Praise for
The One-Day Way

"Empowering, motivating, and inspiring, *The One-Day Way* artfully weaves the story of Chantel Hobbs's weight struggles and triumphs with practical strategies. Chantel shows readers how to change their thoughts and habits to move toward long-term, sustainable weight loss. The key messages—taking each day as it comes and turning negative, sabotaging thoughts into positive ones—are powerful."

—ELISA ZIED, MS, RD, CDN, author of *Nutrition at Your Fingertips* and coauthor of *Feed Your Family Right!*

"*The One-Day Way* shows you how to take your wishes and break them down into achievable goals. Years of bad habits, packing on the pounds, and pursuing an unhealthy lifestyle create huge mountains to climb. *The One-Day Way* makes it possible for you to live life to its fullest throughout your journey to the top!"

—JOSEPH J. TEDESCO, DPT, ATC, CSCS, Elite Physical Therapy, Charlotte, North Carolina

"Chantel Hobbs explores the integral relationship of fitness, food, and faith in a wonderful and provocative way. She shows readers how to incorporate exercise and good nutrition into their everyday lives. I am recommending *The One-Day Way* to all my patients, friends, and family members who have struggled with their weight and who have made the decision to change their lives."

—BARRY ROSS, MD, board-certified gastroenterologist

The One Day Way

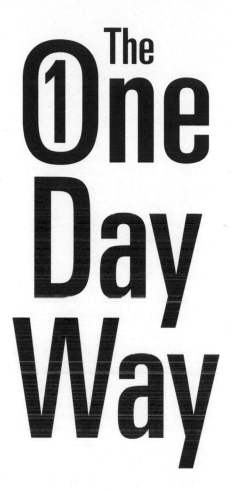

Today Is All the Time You Need to Lose All the Weight You Want

Chantel Hobbs

Author of *Never Say Diet*

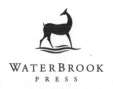

WATERBROOK
PRESS

THE ONE-DAY WAY
PUBLISHED BY WATERBROOK PRESS
12265 Oracle Boulevard, Suite 200
Colorado Springs, Colorado 80921

All Scripture quotations, unless otherwise indicated, are taken from the Holy Bible, New International Version®. NIV®. Copyright © 1973, 1978, 1984 by International Bible Society. Used by permission of Zondervan Publishing House. All rights reserved. Scripture quotations marked (KJV) are taken from the King James Version.

Details in some anecdotes and stories have been changed to protect the identities of the persons involved.

ISBN 978-0-307-45878-0
ISBN 978-0-307-45879-7 (electronic)

Published in the United States by WaterBrook Multnomah, an imprint of the Crown Publishing Group, a division of Random House Inc., New York.

WATERBROOK and its deer colophon are registered trademarks of Random House Inc.

Library of Congress Cataloging-in-Publication Data
Hobbs, Chantel.
   The one-day way : today is all the time you need to lose all the weight you want / Chantel Hobbs. — 1st ed.
      p. cm.
   Includes bibliographical references.
   ISBN 978-0-307-45878-0 — ISBN 978-0-307-45879-7 (electronic)
   1. Weight loss. 2. Weight loss—Psychological aspects. I. Title.
   RM222.2.H5745 2009
   613.2'5—dc22
                                        2009026482

Printed in the United States of America
2009

10 9 8 7 6 5 4 3 2

SPECIAL SALES
Most WaterBrook Multnomah books are available at special quantity discounts when purchased in bulk by corporations, organizations, and special-interest groups. Custom imprinting or excerpting can also be done to fit special needs. For information, please e-mail SpecialMarkets@WaterBrookMultnomah.com or call 1-800-603-7051.

Contents

Part 1: It's Time for Demolition
Leveling the Way You Measure Success

Part 2: Laying the Foundation
One Vision, One Bite-Size Success, One Setback,
One Celebration...at a Time

Part 3: Building the Structure—a New You
Where to Find the Materials, Energy, and Labor for the Project

Part 4: Your Road to Completion
How to Develop Lasting Power

Foreword

I would have benefited from reading *The One-Day Way* when I needed to lose more than one hundred pounds. I never recall setting a goal to be overweight, but years ago I was just that. Growing up in the South, I was raised to believe the preferred way of cooking anything was to first batter it and then deep-fry it. Not the healthiest of options. I finally got to the point where I was sick and tired of always being sick and tired.

In my desire to change my lifestyle, the real issue was not what to do but how to do it. Unfortunately, knowing we have a problem and even being afraid of it doesn't necessarily lead to improved behavior. I had the strongest desire in the world to change, but I thought I had already tried everything, to no avail. I simply did not know how to succeed.

My hope is that by following the wisdom in the pages of this book, you will find the encouragement and knowledge to succeed. The inspiring stories and simple-to-follow meal plans and exercises in *The One-Day Way* can have a real impact on your life. It will help you build new, better habits while making the changes a part of your lifestyle, a part that will become harder to change.

You can start your transformation today, because today is *the day.* Don't try to find time to exercise; *make* the time. Chantel Hobbs touches on all the key aspects of improving your life, especially with her insights into the importance of faith and our inability to make drastic changes on our own.

As Chantel says, "The truth of the One-Day Way is so simple and straight-forward that you might at first discount its power." For your own good, I hope you will read this book to find out.

—MIKE HUCKABEE, marathon runner, host of *Huckabee*,
author of *Quit Digging Your Grave with a Knife and Fork*

For Keith.

You have given me strength and shown me true love in my most desperate hours.

This book exists because of the prayers of a righteous man...

Thank you more than I could ever show or say. I love you, my prince charming.

Acknowledgments

To my daughter Ashley: Your beauty truly radiates from within and attracts many. You are a light in a dark world, so be sure to keep sharing and keep shining.

To my daughter Kayla: Your kindness and willingness to always help amazes me. A heart of compassion and thoughtfulness will always be returned to you when you give without reservation.

To my son Jake: Your spunk and energy for life are contagious. Thank you for making Mommy laugh and always giving me good material.

To my son Luke: Your sweetness and gentleness refresh me daily. Thank you for still letting Mommy sing to you "Night-night, Lukey."

To my mother and father: I can say from the bottom of my heart that you both are experts at living one day at a time! I am eternally grateful for your love, prayers, and support.

To my in-laws, Ken and Linda: Thank you for constantly showing me what true servanthood should look like. I am blessed to know you and have you in my life.

To my dear friends Kerri and Janet: Your prayers, kindness, silliness, and even foot massages will never be forgotten. I hope every other woman in the world may experience the unconditional love and friendship you show me.

To Denise Papaleo (www.denisepapleo.com): I am so grateful you were willing to share your story of victory with my readers. Also, I appreciate your help in creating a fun and challenging One-Day Way workout! Most of all, your friendship is a true blessing.

To Lisa Palmer: Girl, you are dynamite and sugar all rolled into one awesome chick! Our connection was purely a God thing. Keep opening up even when it doesn't seem to make a difference...we won't always be there to see the "after" photo. Just look in the mirror and take yourself back to a long car ride on a Louisiana afternoon. I love you.

To Kelly Hopkins: How you could have missed the finish line for the half marathon at Disney and ended up doing another 13.1 miles (26.2 total) that day is still a mystery to me. But it taught me something about you. You are one determined and tough woman! In this book the readers will understand. You and Tyler have a very special place in my heart.

To Helene: What can I say? A stalker can become a special friend! Your attitude and desire to help spread my message is a testimony of wanting to genuinely change the world by giving people hope.

To Keri White-Kent: Chip was right! You are a sharp and talented woman. Thanks so much for jumping in and helping me pull this project together on a tight deadline.

To Ron Lee: There's no way that having you as my editor has been an accident. Your belief that an author's voice needs to be heard is why God has gifted you to make it sound better. Thank you for a job well done.

Thank you to the entire staff at WaterBrook: From sales to marketing and publicity, you all have a passion for books that can make a difference. Thank you for your genuine enthusiasm for my work.

To my agent, Chip MacGregor: I "get it." Because I do, I want to write books only when I feel I truly have something to say. Thank you for also being a friend.

To the rest of my extended family: I know life can keep us all quite busy. I will always try to be available to you to listen. Just remember, God doesn't need to try; He just is!

To the many people I've met in the past few years who have shared their struggles: Thank you for being so gracious and for trusting me with your deepest pain. You are in my heart and on my mind as I write. Please read this book and recognize that you don't have to let your past hold you back from living life fully *today*!

To the Highest Being: Thank You, Lord, for giving me mercy, especially when I did nothing to deserve it. I pray I will never hesitate to show more mercy to others. Your faithfulness and forgiveness leave me breathless most days. Please help me so that my voice and my words may never be only mine.

· ·

Today Really Can Be Different from the Rest

I'm going to assume you picked up this book because you want to take control of your life so you can lose weight and become healthier. It's probably not the first time you've read a fitness book, and you may be asking yourself, *Can I really do it this time?*

You want to accomplish more than just reaching a lower number on the bathroom scale or being able to say on your Facebook profile, "I work out every day." If you're going to do this, you want it to change your life.

You want to stop revisiting all the issues you can't seem to get a handle on, going back as far as you can remember. But embarking on the adventure of self-improvement, for all the promise it holds, can feel a bit like jumping into an abyss. It's thrilling and scary because you're entering the unknown. You want to break free from the habits that have held you back, but you're beginning to realize that the changes won't last unless you look below the surface. You don't want just another diet; you want to achieve your deepest desires for your life. And you can't do that unless you first look closely at who you really are. It's not easy to take a clear, honest look at yourself, but if you want to experience change that lasts, it's time for you to get beyond that fear.

I have stood at the edge of that abyss. Nine years ago I reached the point where I knew I *had* to change my life. I was so miserable from trying but failing to change that I told myself, for the last time, I would *never* go back to life the way it used to be. I finally lost the weight that had been weighing down my life since childhood. I took off 200 pounds, dropping from nearly 350 pounds. More important, I've kept the weight off. How? I reconstructed more than my body. I rebuilt my entire life, one day at a time, one bite-size goal at a time. I wrote this book to help you do the same thing.

During the years I was overweight, I read so many diet and exercise books that I can't remember them all. Every time I'd pick up a new diet book, I'd hope that finally I was going to discover the secret I'd been searching for. But even as I tried to stir up the ambition to embark on yet another diet, I had an uneasy feeling in the pit of my stomach. Looking back, I know why I had so many doubts. I always knew deep inside that I wasn't ready to do all the things necessary to make permanent changes in my life. I wasn't prepared to look far below the surface to see who I really was and to start changing my life from within.

I know I'm not alone in this. Perhaps you've faced the same fear and it has prevented you from changing your life. The desire to be better, to look better and feel better, is nearly universal. Ask fifty people if they want to improve the quality and intensity of their lives, and overwhelmingly they will answer yes! No one sets a goal to become more frustrated, less healthy, and more miserable next year.

On some level we're all in touch with our inner longing, and most of us want to lose some weight, get in better shape, and regain our confidence. We want to believe in ourselves again. All of these are necessary goals, and they grow out of who we are inside.

So why do so few of us achieve those goals?

WHY OUR GOALS CRUMBLE

In one statement I can show you why your earlier attempts to lose weight and change your life failed. Something in your past convinced you that *this time isn't going to be any different from the rest.* Deep inside, you didn't believe you could change your thinking, your lifestyle, your habits, and your health.

You need to ditch that lie. You really can change, and in dramatic ways, if you will take one crucial step that will solve your lack of confidence. You *can* overcome old habits, old ways of thinking, and past failures by doing one essential thing: *focus on today and today only!*

Your opportunity to change happens today—not yesterday or next week. And your past defeats had little to do with lack of information about how to get fit. If your problem was simply that you didn't know how to diet or the best way to exercise, you could easily solve it by picking up a good nutrition book and an exercise video. The nuts and bolts of healthy eating, exercise, and weight loss are simple: you eat for fuel, you consume fewer calories than you burn, and you exercise for heart health and core strength. We'll spend a few chapters later in this book covering the how-to of weight loss from a practical standpoint.

But before getting into all that, you need to change your mind-set. Most diets fail because the dieter fails to first change the way she thinks. You need to believe differently about yourself, your goals for your life, your health, and the deepest desires of your heart. You need to know there is a way to set and accomplish doable goals and to make them a lasting part of your life. You can change your life, starting today. And only by concentrating on today can you make the changes last.

Your life won't change as a result of setting fantastic and lofty long-range goals. Your life will change because of what you do today and the next day and so on.

I know this contradicts much of what you've read in other books. But that's good news! If the programs you tried in the past produced only temporary success, don't you think it's time to try something completely different? If you're ready to separate from the pack and take the first step in what will be a lasting change in your life, congratulations! You can get started today. And this time really will be different from the past.

WHAT YOU MUST DO BEFORE YOU CHANGE YOUR LIFE

Before I reveal the simple secrets of the One-Day Way of life, I want to mention two things. First, thank you for going on this adventure with me. What I've learned about permanent life change—the things I'll be sharing with you—comes from the deepest place in my heart. Several years ago I crossed a point of no return; I knew there was no turning back. That's when I left behind my old way of living, thinking, and eating. And what I discovered along the way can change your life. (We'll talk more about that in chapter 2).

Second, I know that leaving behind your familiar ways of thinking and living will be uncomfortable, at least at the beginning. I've been there. Entering an adventure such as this one is beautiful and scary, exciting and also deeply personal. It requires that we do this together, and it requires honesty. I promise to be truthful and vulnerable with you, and I need you to commit to letting your guard down as well. Vulnerability is perhaps the greatest key to permanent personal growth. And even if new ways of thinking, eating, exercising, and living start to feel daunting, which they certainly did for me many times, remember we're doing this *together*.

Think Differently, Then Live Differently

If you've ever failed in an attempt to lose weight, you're probably worried that you'll fail yet again. But if you look deep inside, aren't you ready to end the tug of war with the scale and the treadmill? Hopefully, your dreams for the future include not only being healthy and enjoying a maintainable weight but also being a happy and content person and making a positive difference in the lives of others.

Because changing your life is difficult and thinking differently about your life is a challenge, you will be tempted to give up. You'll start thinking that nothing has really changed, and you'll wonder why you're trying to kid yourself. It will be much easier just to go back to your old habits. This is why you need to understand how your thinking always controls your actions. Both negative and positive thoughts have the ability to dictate your actions at any given moment. What gives you the upper hand is that you have a choice: will you make sure that positive thoughts control your mind, or will you give in to negative thoughts? The ability to choose your thoughts and actions gives you tremendous power. You can decide which thoughts will rule your actions, and those decisions will dictate whether you succeed or repeat a past failure.

I guarantee you'll be tempted to give up, so you need to recalibrate your thinking before you try to change your life. Decide right now that you are in this to make a permanent change, no matter the cost. You're not simply trying it out to see if it works. You are trusting that it will work, and you are acting on that belief. *The One-Day Way* will not help you if from the start you already have one foot out the door. It takes full commitment to get full results.

Why You Should Go for It!

I want to tell you one thing that will help you believe it's possible to break old habits, approach your life in a new way, and bring about the changes you've dreamed of. I don't want to sound like I'm giving you a pep talk or delivering a high-school graduation speech. But you must hear this: you *can* change your life in some way, starting today! That's the surprising truth about your life and mine, but it won't help until *you* decide that this time things are going to be different. You have to make a decision that comes from inside. You need to pass the point where going back to old habits, old ways of thinking, and old ways of living is an option.

Changing your life won't always be pretty, but you can do it. And I promise to help you. But I do need one thing from you here at the start: you must believe. I won't ask you to rush out and buy new running shoes, a fancy heart-rate monitor, or a cabinet full of protein powder. All I need from you is will-ingness. That's it. But I'm not talking about casual "I'll give it a try" willingness. This has to be total trust. Trust me as your coach, trust your own ability to commit to the change you desire, and trust the Creator of your mind and body. The God of the universe knows you best, and He wants the best for you.

When I was suffering with my own weight problem, I would look at magazine ads for weight-loss programs and see the "before" and "after" photos. I hated those pictures even though they sometimes enticed me to spend money on the diet system they advertised. I'd cover my eyes, the way a child does while counting in a game of hide-and-seek. You know, pretending not to look while trying to peek through the gaps between my fingers. Seeing the dramatic contrast in the pictures triggered self-loathing. Such a change seemed far beyond my grasp.

So I'm familiar with the hurt you feel deep inside, the hurt that doesn't appear in any "before" photo. Grasping the truth of how to lose weight permanently and gain a new life of passion is a day-to-day process. Losing one pound at a time, strengthening one muscle at a time—that is how you can free yourself from frustration and failure. You're not preparing to embark on a new diet but rather a new way of thinking and living.

The Power of Today

You don't change your life by creating an elaborate flow chart that maps out your fitness program for the next six months. If you want to really change your life, you have to understand that you change it in one day. And that day is today. What you did or failed to do yesterday is in the past. Don't let it drag you down. And what you hope to do tomorrow doesn't matter either. Tomorrow is beyond your reach. What you can control is to choose the best actions today. You change your life with what is immediately in front of you. You have been given today, so use it well.

The truth of the One-Day Way is so simple and straightforward that you might at first discount its power. Here it is: the way to get a new life is to do things today that will propel you to change in small, measurable pieces. Progress is not made in huge steps. It is achieved in bite-size successes. You take a step toward the life you want today, and then another step tomorrow. Getting there is all about making progress from morning to night every day. Don't be interested in perfection; instead be committed to progress.

This time things will be different. Success is not defined by achieving one ultimate goal. With the One-Day Way, success is progress. So you're going to do something you've never done before: you're going to celebrate at the end of each day. Some days you'll celebrate a pound lost; other days it may be that you chose not to grab a candy bar in the grocery checkout line. This is progress, noticeable success, and it's the type of change you can celebrate.

Some days you'll celebrate that you spent an extra fifteen minutes on the treadmill. On other days making it to the parking lot at the gym will be your miracle. Perpetual progress is what moves you toward permanent accomplishments.

The One-Day Way is a system for living life to its fullest. Every day you pursue, without excuses, an irrevocable commitment to optimal health and fitness. That means you will match your decisions to your desire to lose weight, get strong, and live well. Your commitment to a new life will determine your choices from the moment you wake up until you go to bed. Yesterday is irrelevant, and tomorrow is unimportant. Today is what matters, and it is full of all the opportunity you need to be successful.

Before we move on to the specifics of good nutrition, exercise, and weight loss, I advise you first to consult your physician. The nutrition, cardio, and strength-training portions of the One-Day Way are sound, but you should see your personal physician before beginning this or any nutrition, exercise, and fitness program.

I'm glad you're on this journey, and I'm honored to join you. Today we start the biggest adventure of your life. The One-Day Way is not a diet, and it is more than a fitness plan. It is, above all, the path that will lead you to realize your biggest dreams and your deepest longings in life.

Today, things begin to be different.

PART 1

· ·

It's Time
for Demolition

Leveling the Way You Measure Success

. . . .

Chapter 1

Old Habits Are Hard to Break

Let's Make Better Habits That Are Hard to Break Too...

Since we all are creatures of habit, is the person who habitually fails doomed to keep on failing? Even if she wants to change her life, is change impossible?

If you think the answer is yes, I have two more questions for you: Deep down, do you believe you'll always struggle with your weight? Is being overweight your destiny?

It's time to look inside. Have you formed a habit of thinking that contentment and happiness are feelings other people have but you will never experience? Or that success is something only others can achieve? If you've made a habit of thinking this way, then you know that old habits are hard to break—mostly because you've tried for years. But while breaking a habit may be hard, it's not impossible.

I know from experience that counterproductive habits keep us from achieving what we want in life. Like many overweight people, I struggled to improve my life. I'd get on a program and even lose some weight. But as I'd begin to see my body changing, I'd suddenly experience a series of slip-ups. I'm talking a few weekends of wrongdoing, such as indulging in Vegas-style buffet eating while ditching my workouts.

I felt defeated when it came to losing weight. It seemed I couldn't break free from my addiction to food. For as long as I could remember, every time I attempted to overcome the habits that kept me overweight and unhappy, it would end in discouragement and failure. Then I would commit once again to making the necessary changes. I would start getting results, but then I'd let down my guard, pick up a fork, and throw my sneakers in the closet. Not only would I regain the weight I had lost, but I'd also pile on a new load of self-hatred.

Back then, winning never felt possible. In my heart I knew it was just a matter of time before I'd destroy all the progress I'd made. And when that day would inevitably arrive, it felt as if my hard work had been erased. All I would have to show for my efforts were a few more cracks in my already-broken heart. Beyond the pain I felt utterly exhausted thinking about how to regain enough strength to go back to Start.

It's not surprising that I would go months, sometimes years, before trying again to pursue the life I desired.

DESPERATE FOR CHANGE

As I've said, nearly nine years ago my life took a major turn, and I finally won. Truthfully, it required more determination and work than I'd ever devoted to anything else. However, I had reached a point where I could no longer keep living the same way. I was desperate to change, and once I reached that point, I made the commitments necessary to stick with it. After I lost two hundred pounds and became a personal trainer, I knew I had found my new life. And I had to share my experience with the world. I want to convince you that just as I was able to turn my life around after twenty-nine years of constant defeat, so can you.

I can tell you how it happened for me, and I can teach you a nutrition and exercise program that will enable you to lose weight, get healthy, grow strong, and improve your heart health. In fact, we'll do all those things in later chapters. But there is one thing I can't do for you. I can't give you a fearless attitude. And you'll need one if you're going to make permanent changes. You must find it within yourself. If your desire to change is not intense enough to push you past the point of no return, and if you don't have a fearless attitude, you will give up. I'm not being a pessimist; I'm simply speaking from experience.

You and I are the same. I get you, because I am you! I know what it feels like to cross your fingers year after year, hoping and praying that somehow you will finally accomplish this one thing you've set out to do—to lose weight. I understand what it's like to get to the end of your rope once again, so desperate to live a better life that you have trouble breathing some nights as you think about your failures.

While I know your pain, I know freedom as well. I learned things over the past several years that freed me from my prison of self-defeat and self-hate. And in this book I'm going to share them with you. But I can do only so much. You have to be willing to work. I'm not talking about just how to work out but about honest work that will take you to the depths of your soul.

In my work as a personal trainer and life coach, I've known too many people who know what they need to do to get strong and lose weight, yet they can't manage to do it when it gets too challenging. I can talk about good carbs and bad carbs until the cows come home, and it won't do a thing. I can show you new core exercises to make you stronger, but that won't make change happen either. And here's why: to end habitual failure, you have to replace it with habitual success. This means you have to experience it, then repeat the experience again and again. Successes, even small ones, can overshadow your lingering thoughts of inevitable defeat.

So our first goal will be to learn habitual success in a way that doesn't trap you in an overly restrictive program or diet system. You need the freedom to fit the program to your life, goals, and temperament. And since we're concentrating on only one day, you need to be freed from the idea that you measure your success against a pyramid of past triumphs or failures. Most people who are trying to lose weight live in dread of the day they will drop the ball and fail to meet their goals. With the One-Day Way, the only day that counts is today. Keep your past defeats in the past, where they belong.

KEEPING PAST FAILURES AT A SAFE DISTANCE

I was trying to help a woman change her life when I became inspired to create the One-Day Way system. I remember our conversation as if it were yesterday. We sat on a white wicker couch overlooking the Atlantic Ocean. I had counseled and coached this woman, who battled not only a weight problem but also longtime drug addiction. I was so proud of her—she had been living clean, sober, and healthy for 144 days!

But as we sat looking at the ocean, she couldn't see the beauty. All she saw was her pain. She confessed that she had "fallen off the wagon." She was drowning in her failures as she spoke. During our long conversation that afternoon, this tormented soul poured out her heart.

Only days before, she had truly believed she was on the road to freedom, finally. It had been several months since she had stopped letting food and drugs control her life. As she recounted her downward spiral, the details were over-shadowed by a question she was desperate to ask: *How could I have blown 144 days of staying clean, my longest stretch ever, just to end up back in the prison of my addictions?* And truthfully, I was angry and disappointed as well. How *could* she have screwed up again in such a big way? Confessing her failure to me magni-fied her pain, because it meant admitting that she had been concealing her condition, compounding her defeat by hiding it.

After she finished her tragic confession, she asked, "Chantel, am I meant to be like this forever? Can I be fixed, or will I always stay this way?"

For once I had nothing to say. This is not how I roll. I love to hear myself talk, especially when I think I can motivate someone. Yet I found myself think-ing, *Stay this way and do what? Live the rest of your life as an addict?* This was basically what she was implying. *Quickly, Chantel, say something valuable. At least say something to soothe her sadness.* But I had nothing.

For a moment I wondered if she might be right. Perhaps she was going to stay this way. Perhaps she was beyond hope. No. No one is beyond hope. I know firsthand the indescribable feeling of losing weight, reclaiming my life, and breaking free from the addictions that used to keep me trapped! I also know I have nothing that this woman doesn't have. So why did she fail again?

It hit me. She had based her confidence on past accomplishments. Her 144 days of living clean and sober were not her current reality, so dwelling on them wasn't doing her any good. Her life needed to be reconstructed, and I wanted to be the person who would help her create a blueprint for a new life. But first she needed to make her life an active construction site rather than a daily exist-ence of looking backward. Counting up how many days she had fought off her addictions before failing again had done nothing but push her back into despair.

I spoke up and told her, "You can get started on the course of freedom, but it takes something else to stay the course." I knew the truth of the matter because of my own past struggle with addiction and defeat before finally achieving a lasting success.

We live in this world of wanting it our way, now! To our detriment, this has pushed us way off course. We think if we can't achieve tremendous levels of success overnight, then we may as well give up. Rather than giving up, however, we need to change the way we measure success. It has nothing to do with what we accomplished yesterday, even if we accomplished something big for 144 straight days. Instead of focusing on some grand achievement in the past or a distant result in the future, we need to see success as making an irrevocable commitment to live differently. And having made that commitment, we can enjoy success in small quantities while we continue moving forward.

My friend's sense of defeat was compounded by the frustration of breaking her record of 144 days of sobriety. She needed to let go of her past, even her recent past. From now on, I told her, she would have to demolish the way she had been measuring her life—both defeats and victories. She had to stop counting days. It would be great if she could repeat and then exceed her 144 days of sobriety. But having done it once, and even repeating it in the future, would not help her do what she had to do *today* to change her life. She needed to stop worrying about the future, and she needed to let go of the defeat of giving in to her addiction. She needed to realize that what really matters is today.

Someday, somehow, we all are going to fail. The question is whether we will choose to succeed this day, because tomorrow is irrelevant. And our success from yesterday won't change the outcome of what happens today. There is no magical number of successful days that will guarantee a lifetime of success. But if we remove the pressure of trying to make it for a certain length of time and focus instead on living out our commitment for one day, we can reconstruct our lives.

If you want to break an addiction to food, drugs, television, work, a destructive relationship—whatever is keeping you in prison—you will achieve success only by doing it today. This is the basis of the One-Day Way system. You measure success one good decision at a time, one pound at a time, one day at a time as you meet one bite-size goal at a time.

A NEW WAY TO MEASURE SUCCESS

Success has nothing to do with someone else's expectations or your getting into the same size jeans as your best friend wears. The truth is this: success is personal. No one else can dictate how you have to measure your own success. For the woman who has been eating Oreo cookies and potato chips every afternoon for as long as she can remember, going one day without either is a huge deal! That day is a success. Whether or not anyone else struggles with cookies and chips doesn't matter. You'll be amazed how far your small steps, taken consistently, will get you.

The reconstruction of your life starts today. And it will continue in the same way, day by day. One day at a time. Most everything about our lives is broken down into days: our calendars, our work schedules, how long the fish we bought at the grocery store will last before it spoils.

You will build your new life starting with a day. And every day after that you will continue building. At the beginning we'll work together to do a little demolition. We need to clear away the old ways of thinking that have brought you to the point of feeling like a failure. Next we'll create a blueprint, a vision for what you want to look like on the exterior *and* the interior. From there, we will reconstruct your life on three main levels: faith, food, and fitness. You'll learn how to use each one for the best results. And once you have a handle on the One-Day Way system, we'll discuss maintenance and planning for disasters.

The process of taking something that exists and making it better is awesome. Let's get started by building your new mind-set.

. . . .

Chapter 2

Are You at Your Point of No Return?

First Change How You Think

After I told my story of losing two hundred pounds and keeping the weight off in my first book, people started asking me for help.[1] I love using what I've learned about nutrition and exercise to help others reconstruct their lives. But I can only help them when they are truly ready to change.

There is one thing I tell people who say they are desperate: in order to lose weight, live well, and love your life, you first have to reach a point of no return. If you don't pass that point, chances are good that you will eventually return to your old way of living. To make change last, you need to decide that you're not just going to try a diet, but you are going to change your entire lifestyle, *permanently.* Going back to your old life is no longer an option. All permanent life change and personal improvement stem from this decision.

The phrase *point of no return* has a fascinating history. In the first century BC, the Rubicon River stood as a natural boundary between northern and southern Italy, between the province of Gaul and the city of Rome. Because the Rubicon was the border between the two, crossing the river with an army was considered an act of treason.

But on January 10 in 49 BC, Julius Caesar led his troops in crossing the Rubicon in an act of defiance and aggression against Rome. Once he crossed the river, there was no turning back. He had chosen to cross the point of no return, a military move that gave birth to the Roman Empire and eventually affected much of European culture.

The night I crossed my personal point of no return, I knew that things would never be the same again. I was so desperate to change my life that I wouldn't consider any other course of action. I was ready to leave behind my pain and frustration and do whatever was necessary to get fit and achieve a healthy weight. When you reach this point, you make an irrevocable commitment—a decision to press forward and never look back, despite the risks.

What is your personal point of no return? Give it careful thought, because before you can succeed in reconstructing your life, you will have to make some difficult decisions. For your life to truly change—for you to lose all the weight you want and to feel charged up about life—you'll need to cross your own Rubicon.

For me, crossing the line that committed me to living a completely new life was daunting. It meant letting go of things that had provided false security but also were familiar and comforting. It meant changing habits I had developed over twenty-nine years. It meant rethinking some longstanding relationships, both with people and with food. It meant giving up some things I had come to love and learning about new ways of eating and exercising.

Deciding you will charge ahead without ever looking back is the only way you can experience ultimate freedom and victory. There is no other way to leave behind your frustrations and the addictions that hold you back. In the past, temporary success had always left me frustrated and defeated. My life was a series of attempts to apply bandages to seeping wounds. Healing didn't begin until I made a decision never to turn back, to treat the wounds instead of hiding them. You must decide you will never go back to the pain of defeat, no matter how difficult the process may become.

Believe this: whatever you desire, you deserve. Say this one hundred times if you need to. I believe the God of the universe created us to seek more in life and to desire more out of life. He offers us love, peace, joy, well-being, security, and more. And because we are His creation, we deserve His blessings.

The sad reality for many of us is that we sell out our dreams by settling for mediocrity. I know how this happens, because I once was that kind of person. If you believe past mistakes guarantee future failure, stop! You are allowing a lie to prevent you from building a new life. Don't turn your back on joy and happiness—not to mention health and peace of mind. It is possible to change your thinking; it's the only way you'll be able to reconstruct your life.

The point of no return is not a dead end but the beginning of something new—a healthy, meaningful life. Your first one-day commitment is that you vow to *never* return to life the way it used to be.

IT'S TIME TO CROSS YOUR RUBICON

If you lack hope and confidence and feel defeated by past failures, you are the best candidate for enjoying unprecedented success using the One-Day Way system. In fact, you are why I designed it. Crossing the point of no return is your first positive step into a new life that promises an end to counterproductive habits, frustrating setbacks, and discouraging seesaw dieting. As has been said, "It takes one moment to change your attitude, and in that moment, you can change your life."

Other diet and fitness systems tell you to set ambitious goals that you hope to achieve in thirty days, six months, or a year. It's no wonder so many people end up on yo-yo diets and eventually give up entirely. The secret of the One-Day Way is the power you gain from what you think and do right now—not six months from now. You don't win the weight battle in a year. And you won't win it tomorrow. You must choose to be healthy each day.

Don't think about how long it will take to lose the fifteen or fifty pounds you want to take off. Don't try to guess how long it might take you to get really good at exercise. Push those thoughts aside, and in their place take one necessary step that will change your life. To change your life, change the way you think.

It's the first step toward your new life, and you can do it today. You can't build a new life faster than one day at a time, and you start building today with a new way of thinking. Your life can be full of excitement after you pass the point of no return. When you leave behind the barriers and blockades, you'll start accomplishing new goals. And as you achieve things you've been wanting for years, you'll gain a new incentive to achieve even more. Early success feeds greater success later on.

Before long you'll look better and feel better than ever. The by-product will be a surplus of enthusiasm that will keep you moving ahead toward the life you desire, and the enthusiasm will spill over and spread to others. However, before you cross your Rubicon, remember this: "Where there is no vision, the people perish."[2] All the enthusiasm in the world will produce nothing if you don't have a working plan to translate your dreams into reality. As you make an irrevocable decision to lose weight for good, to get fit, and to reconstruct your life, you need an overall picture of what you want to look like. In the following chapter we'll delve further into this.

START BUILDING ON THE INSIDE

If you've ever moved to a different city or decided to look for a home in a new neighborhood, you know that a house's outer appearance often doesn't match what's inside. It's important to think about your own exterior, including a healthy target weight. But before we get there, we're going to start with your interior, and here's why. I've seen homes that look breathtaking, downright picture perfect on the outside. But when you walk inside, you smell a terrible odor or see trash lying around, and the place is total chaos. The conditions inside don't match the beautiful exterior.

We've all met people who look great on the outside but inside are a mess. It's a waste to have it "going on" by a looks-only standard. I've known women with beautiful clothes, the latest hairstyle, and makeup that accentuates their best features, and they still complain constantly about something in their lives. They're never happy. Maybe you've known this kind of person, or perhaps you've *been* this person. You can't hide your unhappiness forever. Eventually the mess inside will start to affect the outside.

If you're not happy with your life, I want you to try this experiment. Stand in a dark room with a candle in one hand and a match or lighter in the other. (As a native South Floridian who's dealt with more hurricane seasons than I can remember, I always have candles and matches on hand.) In the dark of course you can't see. And even when you first light the candle, it will be difficult to see. But as your eyes adjust, you'll see nearly everything that's in the room. If you cared to, you could read or paint your nails.

We all need light to see what's ahead and what's right in front of us. The same is true for your inner life. As you ignite the person you want to be on the inside, you light a fire of passion and purpose. Your reignited inner life will spread light to give you the vision you need to change your outer life.

A New Blueprint for Success

The One-Day Way system will show you how to create a vision and a blueprint that will work especially well with your particular life circumstances, your schedule, and your essential commitments. Whether you're a student, a single mom just trying to get by, a stay-at-home mom, a businessperson, or retired, this is for you! As we begin with the interior, we'll work on your spirit and mind. Then as we transition to your exterior, we'll work on the person you want to see staring back at you in the mirror. This vision is specific. It includes the size you want to wear, how many pounds you need to lose, and what you want your measurements to be. Then I'll help you define the person you want others to see when they meet you. In other words, who is the person you want to put out there to the world?

A big fear many of us face is the fear of repeating past failures. If you made great progress on your last diet and then gained most or all of the weight back, you're frustrated about it. You might be filled with self-doubt, wondering if you can ever make the changes you desire. I receive thousands of e-mails every week, mostly from sad and desperate people. I've learned that the people who tried and failed to keep off their unwanted pounds didn't lack desire. In almost every instance the root problem was their definition of success. Their mind was programmed to define success in terms of a long-range goal, thinking, *If I get to this number by Christmas, I made it.* Success was too far away, which made it seem beyond their reach.

It's no wonder so many people fail at dieting and exercise. None of us can see success a year from now. You can only succeed today. If you desire to create a new life, I will help you attain it—by having daily goals. Because to achieve your goal for tomorrow or next week or next year, you first have to succeed today.

The only reliable measure of success is that you made progress from the day before. If you chose not to eat a cookie today and instead ate a carrot, that's progress. If you chose thirty minutes of exercise rather than putting it off another day, that's success. If this morning you tossed your gym bag into the car so you could exercise on the way home from work, that's success.

The promise of success in the One-Day Way is captured in the word *today*. I didn't name the plan the One-Year Way or even the Ninety-Day Way, since the prospect of doing the right thing for even three months is overwhelming for most people. Let's say you stick to a nutrition and exercise program for even half that time. After forty-five days you're ecstatic! Perhaps in that time you lost several pounds and a few inches. You're doing great. But then, on day forty-six, you look out and notice a Krispy Kreme truck turned over in the street in front of your house. You rush outside to see if you can help, and a doughnut rolls right up to your feet. Suddenly the only toe-touches you do that day are the ones you employ in bending over to pick up free pastries.

After forty-five days of solid discipline, this lapse feels like a major setback. Then on day forty-seven, because you're still so aggravated about the doughnut fiasco the day before, you give in when the pizza delivery man rings your doorbell by mistake. You feel defeated, but you don't need to. If you set out to do *everything* right for six months or even three months, you're virtually guaranteed to fail. No one can do everything exactly right forever. But what if your plan is to do things right for one day? If you've made the commitment, you can stick to your plan and build your new life for a day. And tomorrow you can repeat today's success for one more day. Success builds more success.

The One-Day Way celebrates only the successes of today, so ditch the long-range dieting mind-set, and forget about the hourlong walk a week ago. Instead, shift your focus to the success you can achieve in one day—today. By measuring your successes in a much smaller time frame, you'll see results continuously. And with the encouragement and motivation you'll gain from making daily progress, you'll soon find that you're feeling and looking better than you dreamed was possible!

. . . .

Chapter 3

Don't Run from the Wrecking Ball

You Need to Make Space to Construct a Dream

Imagine you're looking for a new home. You find a house that's situated on a beautiful piece of property right on a beach. You can't get enough of the spectacular views. The beachfront property is roomy enough for a mansion, and you can't believe the shabby, run-down house that sits there. It's too small for your growing family, plus it's poorly constructed. Who would have wasted such a beautiful piece of real estate on this eyesore of a shack?

The house is what real-estate agents refer to as a "tear down." An interested buyer might purchase the property but not to live in the house. The buyer would immediately demolish the structure because it makes more sense to rebuild than to renovate. A new roof or new siding would not transform it into a dream home. So in its place the buyer will build a home that is worthy of the beautiful property it sits on.

Your life is the "house" you live in today. Sometimes all you need is to redecorate a bit or renovate some, but other times you need to tear it down and rebuild something new, strong, and beautiful. And before you start building, you need to demolish your old way of thinking and doing things. You would never build a new structure next to the old, run-down house that came with the land. You'd get rid of the shack to make room for the new. Moving old habits and unhealthy practices out of the way before you start your new life must be the first step toward lasting success.

In the One-Day Way, we start building your new life by getting rid of your old ways of doing and thinking. Certain patterns in your life have kept you defeated and discouraged. These are things you need to change, so let's get rid of them!

GETTING A CLUE ABOUT LOSING WEIGHT

When it comes to losing weight, most people are clueless. I know because I was one of them. In fact, the diet industry banks on our not knowing the facts about weight loss. We choose to believe the myths about fad diets and trendy products that promise to help us lose weight. But when we believe the sales pitch, we're choosing to think in self-defeating ways. We're going to replace self-defeating thinking with something far better!

You've heard the advice to think outside the box. I believe just the opposite: if you want to change your life, you sometimes have to think *inside* the box, or boxes, as the case may be. When my children were toddlers, they loved

Cheerios. After a bit of trial and error (including a lot of spilled Cheerios), I developed a cereal system. When I got home from the grocery story with a new box of cereal, I would open it and pour the contents into separate plastic containers. I had learned by experience that giving a box of Cheerios to a little one sitting in a highchair was not a good idea. Very few pieces of cereal made it into the child's mouth.

I realized the best way to let my children enjoy all the Cheerios was to put the cereal into smaller containers. A toddler can handle a small container of cereal and not make a huge mess. And he gets to enjoy even more of his crunchy, gum-soothing treat.

Whenever we break big things into smaller pieces, or put our big goals into smaller boxes, in the long run we are able to grab hold of more of the big thing we desire. Less of it gets lost in the process. When you take the time to break down a huge goal—such as changing your life—into little "containers," the task suddenly becomes doable.

Change takes time, and when a goal is set for long-range progress, it can seem so far away that you get discouraged before you start making progress. Dieting experts and even goal-setting gurus have had little effect on helping us lose weight or make other major changes in our lives because they hand us too big a box. Much of the popular thinking is to do everything bigger and better and on a grand scale. It's the think-outside-the-box mentality. But I believe this type of thinking usually gets us off track. So with the One-Day Way, rather than encouraging you to dream big, I want you to start by dreaming small—in bite-size pieces. But know this: big dreams are still coming true. If you break your dreams down into doable pieces, you'll make noticeable progress every day. You'll be encouraged and inspired by your progress rather than being overwhelmed by a huge, six-month plan.

And the best part is this: when you gradually get to and through a big box (or big goals, in this case) by breaking it down into bite-size steps, you've had just enough to make you want more! Taking small steps is the key to moving forward and bringing about lasting change. You'll have more success in accomplishing your long-range goals if you will break them down into small boxes.

ACHIEVING A BIGGER DREAM

I'm not suggesting that you limit your dreams. I have huge dreams, and I know you have too. When I decided at age twenty-nine that I was done with being two hundred pounds overweight and ready to build a completely new life, that dream was huge. You want a new life too. Doing what it takes to turn a dream that size into reality is not for the faint of heart.

It gets done not in huge leaps but in doable steps. It's easier to open a jewelry box than a bank vault, right? Most people try to put their dreams into a giant container, assuming that a big dream calls for enormous goals. But we fail to realize that oversize goals don't fit into a normal life, so they end up getting set aside. That's why so many of us feel defeated.

So let's demolish the big-box thinking. We'll do it by discovering a new way to measure success. From now on you're going to measure success based on small, attainable goals. Begin each morning thinking about a few things you can do that day that will bring you closer to accomplishing something bigger. When it comes to weight loss, today's success might be adding intensity to a workout or saying no to the french fries that come with lunch. As you achieve small goals, you'll have reasons to celebrate every day. Think about attending a party that is such a blast you don't want it to end. That's the feeling you can enjoy every day as your small successes lead to more and greater success.

The second kind of thinking we need to demolish is comparing. All our lives we've learned to compete and compare. We are constantly comparing ourselves to others, which hurts our relationships and our self-esteem. It seems to be ingrained in everyone, even young children. I can't count how many times I've made ice cream sundaes for my kids only to hear whining! Instead of "Wow, this looks yummy," I hear "Why does he get more chocolate syrup and whipped cream than me?" My kids can miss the joy of eating ice cream because they're focused on what they don't have.

When you visit a friend's new home, it's natural to compare it to yours. Is it bigger? Are the furnishings nicer? We compare our looks, our size, our clothes. We feel inferior or sometimes superior, based not on our intrinsic value but on how we think we stack up against the competition. This kind of thinking hurts us, and it prevents us from changing our lives.

For you to succeed in changing your life, you have to shift your focus away from making comparisons with others and concentrate on making progress toward your goals. If you're doing this only to compete with someone else, you'll stay miserable. So if you've been dreaming of the day you'll fit into a dress size that matches what your best friend wears, get over it. Don't try to change your life to impress a friend or to compete against anyone. If that is your main goal, you won't be satisfied when you get there. You'll only find some other way you don't measure up. Then you'll set another goal, based on a new comparison with a friend who is even thinner or taller, younger, stronger. It never stops, so don't even start. There will always be someone thinner than you with better hair and a more stylish wardrobe. If you're motivated only by someone else's life, you'll never feel good about your own.

Before you can reconstruct your life, you have to demolish these two ways of thinking. Stop telling yourself you have to accomplish huge goals, and stop comparing yourself with anyone other than yourself. To demolish the first habit, break big goals down into doable steps. To knock down the second one, decide to compare yourself only to yourself. You can compare your life today with your life yesterday or the day before. That's how you measure personal success.

TAKE A COMPLETELY DIFFERENT ROUTE

Losing weight and getting fit one day at a time will require you to rethink many of the standard routes you used to take in the past. You can't revolutionize your life if you take the same road that last time led to frustration.

Although the word *maverick* was overused during the 2008 presidential campaign, I loved hearing it applied to John McCain. To me, a maverick is someone who goes to great lengths, no matter what anyone else thinks or says, to get a job done. A maverick doesn't compare himself to others or try to please the rule makers. He follows his own vision. This is the attitude we all need, not in a political sense, but as we seek to build a new life.

If you learn to think like a maverick, you'll approach weight loss differently than you've done before. You'll accept that losing weight has nothing to do with good genes and says nothing about your worth as an individual. It's all about math. You take in fewer calories than you burn. As you do this over time, you lose pounds. That's pretty much it.

What if you woke up every day and thought, *I must work out today and eat a little less so my body will use some excess fat to keep me going*? Instead of obsessing about points or calories or how much and how often you'll work out, you are simply opening a small box. In order to make the math work (burn more calories than you consume), you decide to break a sweat. By exerting your body, you burn calories. That's just one small box, and it's one you can easily open today. Tomorrow you'll open another box. But you're not thinking about tomorrow. Today you concentrate on today's small box by breaking a sweat.

And what about opening small boxes when it comes to food choices? Maybe your bite-size goal for today is to pass up the second cookie and all the potato chips. You say no to junk food. As you do that today, you can begin to visualize the fat on your thighs shrinking. And hopefully that's a powerful-enough image that you'll decide to open another small box: a decision to eat more vegetables and less pasta at dinner. Or you might open a small box that involves eating fresh fruit instead of candy for a snack.

These might seem like insignificant steps. But that's where you have to stop comparing. To make this work, you have to embrace the revolutionary idea that the small, bite-size choices you make today will make a big difference in your life. At the end of the day, you realize you took a small step, or a few steps, toward being healthy. Tomorrow there will be another opportunity to break a sweat and make good choices about what you eat. Before too long you will look as good as you feel.

You never need to worry about long-term meal plans and fancy workout strategies. The simplicity of the One-Day Way program grows out of the idea that what you did yesterday doesn't really matter. It plays no part in your actions and choices for today. With each new day you have new choices to make and more chances to make the right choices. Every day you take advantage of a new opportunity to live well and be your best.

This system offers you an unexpected bonus: if you make a mistake, you can forgive yourself, because each day is a new start. Maybe you slipped up yesterday, but that was yesterday. It's history. Eating one cookie isn't such a tragedy that it will trigger a cookie binge because you're feeling guilty about having failed. Each new day you start again to make one healthy choice at a time.

Have you ever imagined how a person released from prison must feel? It must be an overwhelming feeling to be given the chance to start over again. That's the feeling I want you to wake up with every morning. You're getting another chance to escape the jail of self-defeating habits and to feel good about your life. Don't worry about what happened yesterday or even about long-term goals. Your goal for today is doable, and achieving it will fuel more achievements tomorrow. That's all part of thinking inside the box.

Get rid of the feeling that by now you should be further along or that you need a magic pill to fix everything. Wherever you are today, that's where you'll start. And there is no magic pill. It's up to you to change your life, and you can do it!

Tear down the habits that work against you—a tendency to set huge goals, the habit of comparing yourself to others, and the temptation to measure success in ways that are self-defeating. When you demolish these habits, you'll have cleared enough space to start building your new life.

Chapter 4

The Power of One Day

Building a New Life
Only Takes One Day

It's easy to assume that your efforts to change your life don't really count until you lose a specific amount of weight or fit into a certain size or even hit the gym for a solid month. But when you think in those terms, what happens if you miss your goal of losing ten pounds? Or how do you handle it if you miss two days at the gym, even after you've been there every day for three straight weeks?

When you define success as the achievement of long-range goals, you're bound to feel like a failure sooner or later. Instead of celebrating the many steps you're taking toward permanent life change, you beat yourself up because you have "failed." That's why most people don't stick with a diet or a fitness system. They don't make the quick progress they'd hoped for, so they get discouraged and give up.

You need to discard that way of thinking. The One-Day Way focuses your efforts and your celebrations on one day: today. With this system you don't succeed by lowering your standards. It's just the opposite. Instead of going on a diet for a few months, you change your entire lifestyle, one day at a time. The One-Day Way redefines the way you measure success, and it incorporates regular celebrations along the way. As you work this program, you'll learn to let go of unrealistic, self-defeating goals. Instead, you'll embrace the desire to be your best every day. That is your goal for today and every day.

The main objective is not just to lose weight but to keep it off. I'll show you how to stop the cycle of losing and gaining and start a pattern of healthy living. Have you ever noticed that when a building is under construction, people stop to look? They're trying to figure out what's being built. With the One-Day Way system, what's being built is your new life of purpose and passion—as well as your newly fit and healthy body.

Every building needs a foundation. You don't start building a house by hanging the curtains or putting on the roof. Those tasks come later. You first have to fit together the materials for the foundation, or else everything after that will fall apart. The strength and quality of a building lie in the things you can't see from the outside—the foundation and framework. Likewise, as you begin building your new lifestyle, you need to begin with a solid foundation.

When my sons were little, they enjoyed playing with wooden Lincoln Logs. At the age of three, my youngest, Luke, didn't understand how to stack the toy logs in alternating directions. One afternoon he sat on the floor and stacked the logs parallel to one another. Without the balance created by criss-crossing and interlocking the logs, the structure collapsed, and logs scattered. A typical toddler, Luke responded with tears and a tantrum, but it gave me the chance to show him how to start over. I taught him how to arrange the logs to make his house both big and strong.

Can you relate to Luke's attempt to build with Lincoln Logs? Have you ever had a vision for what you wanted your life to become, but then you grew impatient with the process? Has achieving a big goal over several months become such a far-off dream that you got discouraged and quit after a few months? Or maybe after just four or five weeks? Most of us don't have the patience, the perseverance, or the ironclad willpower to set a goal for a year or half a year and then reorganize our entire lives to accomplish that goal. But like my young son with his Lincoln Logs, we can learn to identify the building blocks and understand how they fit together.

Building the foundation of your new life involves a very simple process. You do what is needed today without thinking about tomorrow or next week. Your entire responsibility is to work on the appropriate building blocks for today. You don't worry if you're on pace to achieve a six-month goal. You don't lose your focus by wondering if the system is even working. Instead, you trust the process. And tomorrow you repeat the process. After six months of working on the building blocks for one day, you'll find that you have built a life that is very different from the one you started with. And amazingly, your new life will look a lot like the one you've dreamed of for years.

FOCUSING ON FAITH, FOOD, AND FITNESS

As you begin work on the foundation of your new life, you need to change the way you think about achievement, the way you think about setbacks, and the way you think about getting through each day. Practicing the One-Day Way of life changes the way you look at three things: faith, food, and fitness. If you're ready to lose weight for good and rebuild your life, these three building materials are essential. Each one must be solid and strong, or the whole thing could easily collapse. Many people try to lose weight simply by changing their eating habits for a short time. But they come at their program with a "maybe" attitude instead of faith. And they don't reinforce their dietary changes with steps toward greater fitness. Pretty soon, without the combination of faith, food, and fitness, things fall apart.

We'll talk more in part 3 about the specific steps you'll take to reconstruct your life. For now, give serious thought to the three essential components of the One-Day Way.

Faith

The One-Day Way is based on having faith (and I'm not talking about being religious). Faith is simply having a firm belief in something that hasn't been proven beyond all doubt. That belief is what makes things happen. Every accomplishment in your life, every risk you take, everything that you believe in and fight for is based on some level of faith.

The quest for all self-improvement is built on a form of faith. If you don't believe the One-Day Way will help you, it probably won't, because you won't make an irrevocable commitment to it. You can't build a new life on a foundation of skepticism. But if you have even a little bit of faith, it can grow.

You've seen it happen before: you become what you believe. When you believe you are destined to live a defeated life, you give in to defeat. To change your life, you have to believe differently. If you believe you'll always struggle with being overweight, hating to exercise, and giving in to your food cravings, you're not living in faith. Faith says the opposite. It says you are meant for more, for a life that brings joy and fulfillment. You are meant to have a life that makes you the victor and not the victim.

Having faith means you will combat the forces that work against you at all costs. Your friends and family may not be as encouraging as you would like. And your past failures will try to haunt you and to steal your new life. So you must decide now that you will believe in your reconstruction project *no matter what.*

You might be thinking, *I really don't know if I have the faith in myself to do this. I really don't know if I believe in the One-Day Way.* That's okay. As you celebrate each small step, your faith will grow. Every day you'll take action, and most days you'll experience results. That is what will make your faith grow.

Food

Next I want you to think about your relationship with food. Specifically, does food control you, or do you control your food?

Over the years as I tried to lose weight, different people told me I had to learn to "eat to live rather than live to eat." In other words, I had to view food simply as the necessary fuel to keep me alive, like gasoline for a car. I had to move from obsessing about food to being sort of bored by it in order to take away its emotional power over my life.

The thing is, I don't buy into this idea 100 percent of the time. Yes, food is primarily fuel. Yes, food should not exercise emotional power over us on a regular basis. But food should also be enjoyed. I've revamped some of my thinking about food as I've continued to maintain a healthy weight for nearly a decade.

Here is the best way to develop a healthy relationship with food. On most days select the food you eat based on its being fuel, not a friend. You need it to live, and you want to put the best-quality fuel into your body. And you must control the amount of food you eat if you want to lose weight.

In chapter 13 you'll find detailed sample meal plans that spell out what to eat and how much so you can lose weight. But as you do this, you also need to plan for times when pleasure can and should come from eating. If you're planning to attend a birthday party, you might want to join the celebration by having a piece (not three) of cake. Go ahead and enjoy the fun of tasting something yummy!

If you've abused food in the past, you might think it's the enemy. But that type of thinking assumes that food has power, and you can end up feeling as if you have no control over it. Food addiction is unlike dependence on alcohol or drugs. Alcoholics and drug addicts can control their addiction through total abstinence. But you can't rid yourself of a food addiction by giving up food altogether. So you need to take control. One day at a time you'll begin to re-connect with food in a healthy way. You'll no longer give food the power to control your mind.

A big part of regaining control over food is developing a healthy balance in your view of it. The temptation to gorge will lessen as you learn to enjoy food without abusing it. Knowing in advance that you can enjoy delicious food at the right time (but not all the time) will keep you from feeling deprived. If you know you have the freedom to eat, it becomes less a temptation and more a matter of good planning. Your food guilt will be a thing of the past. No more self-sabotaging.

Food is the building material you need for reconstructing your body in a healthy way, so realize you need to cultivate the proper attitude toward it.

Fitness

Finally, let's talk about fitness. Our bodies weren't made just to sit around. They are wonderfully complex machines that were designed to move. We can't be at our best without regular exercise to strengthen our hearts and develop core fitness.

I recently had to be in New York for work, and I was reminded of how amazing our bodies are. I would normally never choose to be in New York in winter. I'm a beach girl who loves sunshine and warm temperatures. Living in southern Florida my entire life has also kept my blood thin. (I have even envisioned hell as a really cold place instead of a hot one.) So you can understand the misery I felt on that dreary, freezing day in Manhattan.

A Daily Reminder

Unless you're the world's most organized person, a visual reminder is helpful. As you work on reconstructing your life, check my Web site (www.chantelhobbs.com) and get the One-Day Way bracelet. This can be your daily reminder that you're building a new life.

One side simply reads "One-Day Way." This will remind you to make the best choices you can today—using faith, food, and fitness.

The other side of the bracelet reads "Tomorrow's almost here!" You'll flip it to that side for one of two reasons. First, when you feel like you've blown it, flip it as a reminder that in the morning you'll have a fresh start. This will help you not to give up. Second, you can flip to the "tomorrow" side at the end of the day as you assess how it went. The following morning, as you recommit to being the best you can be, you'll flip it back to the One-Day Way side.

I had a meeting to go to, and since it was only a few blocks from my hotel, I decided to walk. But I was bundled up so much it was hard to move. I was wearing two scarves, a few layers of sweaters, a coat, and a hat. The only thing missing was gloves, because I forgot to pack them. As I began my winter trek, I put my hands deep in my coat pockets to keep them warm. But having my arms plastered to my sides slowed me down. I was already running late for the meeting, and with my arms immobilized, my legs couldn't move very fast. Desperate, I pulled my hands out and began to swing my arms. Suddenly I was cruising along much faster (and getting a little warmer). Moving my arms and legs together created power—a serious synergy was taking place.

Your body was designed to move! And the bonus is that when you expend energy to move, you get *more* energy. It's counterintuitive but true. Learning the necessity of regular movement will change your outlook on fitness. You can stop dreading exercise when you understand you are designed to do it. (And no one expects you to become a bodybuilder or a marathon runner, unless you find that's what you want to do.)

As you start moving every day, you'll begin to like it more. Then you'll like it a lot, and then you'll very likely love it. The day will come when you're unable to get outside or to the gym to work out, and you'll be *disappointed*.

I began my personal program at age twenty-nine, not by dieting, but by exercising every day. Remember, I once weighed 350 pounds. When I set out to change my life, I didn't just lose 200 pounds. I ended up building a new life that includes good nutrition and regular exercise. I achieved my target weight and, in the process, became strong. It's a little crazy to think I've run several marathons and trained other runners for marathons. How? Because a marathon is finished one mile at a time. Running 26.2 miles seems insane, but I know firsthand it's possible.

As I've said, you and I were made to move; our bodies are not designed to be stationary. In the process of building your new life with the One-Day Way system, you'll love getting stronger, more toned, more fit. In later chapters I'll show you simple ways to make exercise fun. You won't need an expensive gym membership, you won't need to spend your whole day working out, and you won't have to train for a marathon. But you will have to commit to movement, to using your body to do what it was designed to do.

A New Life That Lasts

By changing the way you think about faith, food, and fitness, you will reconstruct your life. You will lose weight and keep it off forever, which requires commitment and self-discipline. But discipline is not a bad thing. If you hire people to build a house, don't you want them to be disciplined as they build it?

The pain of regret can be far worse than the pain of discipline. Discipline is not punishment; it is shaping the way you live. In time you'll value discipline because it gives you freedom—the freedom to be healthy, strong, and happy. With the One-Day Way system, you'll develop discipline day by day instead of worrying about the "bigness" of your long-term goals. You'll focus on today rather than on a month from now or a year from now.

In the next several chapters, you'll start drawing up some plans. You'll accurately assess your strengths and determine what you want to change. As the architect of your new life, you'll decide what you want to build. You have the power within you to be remarkable, to lose the weight that has been weighing you down, and to feel alive and full of more energy than you can contain.

Lisa's One-Day Way Story

I've struggled with obesity since childhood. I learned early how delicious food could be, and I wouldn't stop eating until I felt sick. I grew up thinking that feeling sick meant my stomach was full. Thus began an unhealthy relationship with food.

By the time I was in tenth grade, I weighed about 245 pounds. A few years later, when I met the man of my dreams, I felt there was no way I would ever have a chance with him. But he looked beyond my external appearance and appreciated the real me.

Getting married is supposed to be the happiest time in a girl's life, but for me there was sadness as well. I had to pick between two dresses, the only ones in my size (24). When my dress came in, I went to try it on and found that it was too small. The seamstress had to add extra material to the back so it would fit. I was mortified.

The day I got married, I weighed about 270 pounds. As I walked down the aisle, I saw my soon-to-be husband beaming. I couldn't understand why he was happy, because in that moment I was embarrassed for him.

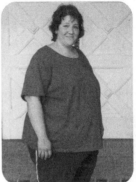

Photo by David Palmer

During the first years of our marriage, there were many times when I broke down and cried over my weight. But despite my frustration, I didn't lose any weight. In fact, in that first year I gained about 25 pounds. I know what it's like to walk into a restaurant and feel everyone staring. I could feel their condemnation. I know what it's like to scan the room for a chair that I could fit in instead of choosing to sit in a booth. But even those things didn't prepare me for what I experienced the day I gave birth to my son.

They wheeled me in for a cesarean section. This was my first child, and I was nervous. When the time came for them to begin the surgery, I heard a noise that sounded like duct tape being ripped. They were taping the fat on my stomach to pull it up so the doctor could see how to cut the baby out. I wanted to disappear. I had a healthy baby boy, but the emotional scars of that moment would last a long time.

Two years later we had a beautiful baby girl. I had a good life with a husband who loved me, but I still had such intense sadness inside. On some nights I would cry myself to sleep, feeling hopeless. But then I'd stuff the feelings back down, trying to ignore them.

In 2006 my sister-in-law asked me to start working out with her and a group of women at my mother's home. I worked out with the group for about a year, but I didn't lose any weight. I reasoned that because I was working out, I could eat whatever I wanted.

Then a woman I knew mentioned that she wanted to put on a weight-loss seminar. She was looking for someone who would come speak. I told her that my cousin's wife, Chantel Hobbs, had lost 200 pounds and was writing a book. The week before Chantel came to speak at the seminar, I had applied for health and life insurance and was denied. It felt like all the air had been sucked out of me.

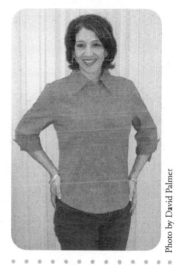

Chantel flew in on a Friday. My mother, my sister-in-law, and I took her to lunch. I will never forget how hopeless I felt when I put the car in reverse and she looked at me and said, "Lisa, I think I made this trip just for you." The next thirty minutes began to change my life. Chantel said things I had never heard. She told me about many of the things you've been reading in this book.

Photo by David Palmer

I couldn't wrap my brain around the fact that it could be as simple as making healthy choices one day at a time. After the seminar ended, Chantel was preparing to fly back home. She told me, "It's already in you! Just trust yourself. You can do this."

The next day I awoke to a 180-pound mountain staring me in the face. That was how much weight I wanted to lose. I didn't know how or even if I could do it. But I knew I was going to give it my all. That's when I began thinking differently. No matter how many times I messed up, I was not going to quit. One day at time, one meal at a time. I gave myself no option to fail.

This awesome journey started on February 1, 2007. All the things Chantel had told me kept playing over and over in my mind. By April I had lost nearly 40 pounds. By August, I had lost 80 pounds. And by Thanksgiving I had hit the 100-pound mark. I was not going to stop until I got to where I wanted to be!

In October 2008 I reached my goal of losing 180 pounds! The time went so quickly when I focused on one day at a time. I woke up every day and embraced that day, doing the work for one day.

My husband and kids have been my biggest cheerleaders! I've kept the weight off for more than two years, but they tell me they can't remember me when I was "big." I now realize that during all those years of wanting to lose weight and to feel normal, it was right there in front of me. I just couldn't see it because I let my mind get in the way.

Today I have so much joy! I feel like I am finally the person God created me to be. I now co-lead a weight-loss group at my church, and I'm a much happier wife and mother. Anyone can do this, even people like me who used to hate to exercise. You do it just as Chantel says—one day at a time.

. . . .

Chapter 5

Letting the Dust Settle

The One-Day Way Fast

Once we demolish negative habits, a bit of cleanup is required before your new construction can begin. Believe it or not, I need you to stop and let the dust settle before starting work on a new life.

By now I hope you've basically demolished your old ways of thinking (although you may still need to work on the demolition a little bit every day). I hope you're thinking in terms of bite-site celebrations each day. You're working toward weight loss and improved fitness and health, and you've begun to think how to put your large goals into smaller boxes.

In chapter 3 we looked at some of the daily decisions you need to make to succeed with the One-Day

Way system. You will no longer compare yourself to others, you will measure progress by making and meeting daily goals, and you will trust that achieving small successes will propel you forward. By freeing yourself from self-defeating thinking and by breaking your goals into bite-size pieces, you will establish a pattern for lasting weight loss and fitness. However, old habits and ways of thinking won't go away easily. There will be times when you won't feel content with your progress. You'll get frustrated and wish you could see major results and see them *now*!

But before we move forward, I want to share an essential component of the One-Day Way. Successful life reconstruction depends on letting the dust settle for a day before you break ground on your new life. After demolition is complete, if the workers rushed back in and began to rebuild, they'd be working in a cloud of dust. As this pertains to building your new life, I feel the best way to allow the dust to settle is to fast for one day.

Fasting is an ancient practice that is gaining new prominence. It involves going without food for a specified time. I can guess what you're thinking—a *whole day* without food? Actually, thinking about it is harder than doing it. So don't think about deprivation; think about the benefits of delaying gratification for a day. You are choosing to fast, you are making it doable by deciding in advance that it's just for one day, and afterward you can celebrate the success of having done the thing you chose to accomplish.

I have to tell you, fasting is the greatest thing I've ever found to clear my mind and help me focus. I can't make you do this, and I imagine you might feel tempted to skip this chapter. But this simple exercise is a great way to begin your new way of thinking, which will lead to building your new life. If you're serious about your goals, make use of this powerful tool. (And if you're still on the fence, perhaps you're just not quite ready to change your life.)

Notice that I didn't say fasting is the greatest way to lose weight. Rather it's a practice that helps you focus. The One-Day Way is designed to help you change your entire life, not simply to lose weight and get fit. I want you also to gain spiritual strength. The strength I'm talking about doesn't come from joining a religion. If you're overweight, you already know that it's not solely a physical problem. It affects you emotionally and spiritually as well. Spiritual strength will enhance your physical strength.

Perhaps you're thinking, *I'm not that into spiritual stuff.* That doesn't matter. Every one of us is spiritual—it's part of who you are just as much as your physical being. Without a balance of the mind, body, and spirit working together, life feels out of whack.

CLEAR YOUR MIND, GAIN GREATER FOCUS

The self-sacrifice involved in giving up something, whether it's eating the wrong foods or watching too much television or working late too often, makes you more aware of your values and priorities. When you give up food during a fast, it leads to emotional, physical, and spiritual clarity. It's a way to cleanse your body and mind, allowing the dust to settle.

Over the past several years, I have worked with a variety of people as their personal trainer. Among my clients are Jewish women who celebrate all the traditional holidays. While some holidays involve feasts, others call for fasting. I'm always fascinated by the way my clients find clarity and spiritual renewal in fasting.

Interestingly, many Jews give up yeast during Passover, eating unleavened bread instead. And in doing this they celebrate God's deliverance of their ancestors from slavery in Egypt. (This is the story of the Exodus in the Bible.) Because the Israelite slaves left Egypt so quickly, they didn't have time to let the bread rise. So today when Jews eat unleavened bread at Passover, they aren't depriving themselves but are celebrating a miracle of deliverance. It's a time to focus on the beauty of freedom, a gift they now enjoy, and not a time to focus on what they're giving up.

I've often fasted when I was facing a big decision or was about to do something hard and knew I didn't have the strength. The clarity and emotional power I gain from fasting is life changing. I think you'll find this to be true in your life as well. If you're serious about overhauling your body and other areas of your life, then a twenty-four-hour period without food will be extremely beneficial.

Denying our desires translates into sharper thinking. When we struggle with our weight, we often think that our desires are stronger than we are or that we're victims of the whims of our appetites. You are stronger than that! And even if you're not sure you believe it, it's time to start living as though you believe it. When you fast for just one day, you realize how capable you are. You learn that you don't have to be a victim.

If you're resisting the idea of a fast, you're not alone. Whenever I suggest this to people, almost always they come up with an excuse. "You don't understand my job. I couldn't work and not eat for a day." Or "I'm planning to go to a party that night." When I suggest they fast on another day, they suddenly remember there's another party that night as well...

Food is important to us. It's the center of most social occasions, and it's the tasty break we get in the middle of the day. It has emotional meaning as well. But know this. A fast can help put food in perspective. We can get by for one day without it. And don't worry that you'll wreck your metabolism in twenty-four hours. If food occupies too much of your thinking and planning, this one day will be a chance to reprioritize and to break the power food has over your life.

My daughter Ashley recently completed her first fast. She wasn't fasting to lose weight but rather to support a friend. How cool is that? Her closest friend was preparing for a missions trip to Ethiopia. Those going on the trip devoted one day to eating nothing but rice in order to experience the typical diet of Ethiopians. Even though Ashley wasn't going on the trip, she wanted to support and pray for her friend. She also wanted to feel some of what it would be like to live in a third-world country for a day.

The night before her fast, Ashley cooked a pot of brown rice and put it into three small containers: one for breakfast, one for lunch, and one for dinner. Later that day she sent me a text message from school. In it she said, "I'm starving!" A little while later she sent another text: "Brown rice is disgusting." I laughed when I read them, and I found myself smiling all day. I was so proud of her. I realized the value of her commitment and the potential long-lasting effect of it. My beautiful daughter would learn on this day that self-sacrifice can offer something that regular indulgence can never deliver.

Not giving in to familiar desires creates a shift in what you desire. There is a resourcefulness that comes from giving up something important. As Ashley feasted on brown rice all day instead of eating her usual bagel, peanut butter and jelly sandwich, and chips, she could think more about the Ethiopian way of life. She chose to shift her focus from her own hunger to the pain of the people her friend would be helping. She realized that what she endured for one day, many people around the world endure every day. That opened a new place of empathy and compassion in her heart.

GETTING THE MOST FROM YOUR FAST

Fasting requires a small bit of preparation. The day before, you might be tempted to overeat to compensate. If you do that, it will make fasting more difficult. So instead of eating a pint of ice cream and a slab of ribs the night before, drink plenty of water. Eat lots of fresh fruits and vegetables. This will ensure a good supply of quality energy for the day. You'll still feel hungry, of course, and that's part of the value of the fast. You'll realize that even if you feel hungry, you'll survive.

Begin your fast day with gratitude. Make a list of your blessings. Focus on them throughout the day. In fact, try to think of some that are not so obvious, such as a person who rubs you the wrong way. The blessing is that because you have this person in your life, you've developed more patience and greater understanding. Consider this day as the beginning of a special journey in which you will gain new insights and see things more clearly. Learning to let go of yesterday and live in the moment will reap unexpected rewards.

Also remember that fasting is part of cleansing the body. When your body uses up all the converted food that's available and still needs more energy, it will begin to tap into other places. Places it doesn't go to very often, mostly because it is fed so regularly it doesn't need to. During a fast your body will be working hard to keep everything running smoothly. You will be tapping into your body's reserves. After a period of fasting, miraculously your energy levels also improve because you're not bogged down with the chemicals and junk from so many of the foods we put in our bodies.

Your brain is another story. When you go without the nourishment your brain is accustomed to, initially you may feel sluggish. Don't give up though, because in a short time your senses will become heightened. Without the chemical releases that come from food, your mind is more keenly aware of many other sources of energy. For example, breathing deeply can provide your body with energy. Also, on a practical level, when you're freed from thinking about what to eat next, you can focus on other things. You'll find you have time to think about your goals and how you can begin to break them into bite-size steps. You'll become more resourceful than ever before.

Throughout the day continue to remind yourself that you are blessed to live in a land of plenty. It is no small blessing that sacrificing food is something you can choose, not something you are forced to do. When you go without food, you realize more than ever that food is given to us for energy first and pleasure second. Food is fuel to keep our bodies working. As you go without nourishment for one day, give some thought to whether you've misused food—as comfort or as a drug or as a friend—rather than fuel. Be open to the new insights that going without food can bring.

Once you're in the full swing of the One-Day Way, you should fast one meal once a week. That is, you skip one meal every week. Be sure to drink plenty of water to stay hydrated. And be sure you don't overeat prior to the one-meal fast or at the following meal to compensate. Rather, use the weekly fast to regain your perspective, to check the attitude of your mind and heart.

As you give up food on a regular basis, you continue to send your body and your brain the message that food will no longer control your life. Instead, you're controlling when to celebrate with food and when to sacrifice by skipping food.

A fasting lifestyle may eventually take on much more meaning in your life. The powerful feeling of resisting temptation can be habit forming. It may be that food is your greatest temptation, but you also can fast from other things. Anytime you realize that something (a hobby, a recreational pursuit, a person) is beginning to control you, consider fasting from that activity or relationship. Some people choose to fast from television, from surfing the Internet, or even from buying gossip magazines in the supermarket checkout line!

One week I even chose to give up exercise. For me, to fast from exercise was more difficult than giving up any food could ever be. I found myself trying to exercise using the goofiest stuff, like doing biceps curls with canned goods while grocery shopping. I was trying to get the endorphin high. Then it dawned on me: I was cheating. The endorphins were precisely what I was becoming too dependent on and what I needed to fast from.

Fasting is a tool you can use to find freedom. Begin with the one-day fast. Next try the regular weekly fast from one meal. Inner strength can come from working to give up something just as much as it can from working to get what you want.

. . . .

PART 2

Laying the Foundation

One Vision, One Bite-Size Success, One Setback, One Celebration...at a Time

Chapter 6

You Are Now the Architect of Your Life

It's Time to Decide What You Want to Build

If there's one thing I've learned in my work with people of many different shapes and sizes, it's that different people want to achieve different things. Not only is beauty in the eye of the beholder; beauty comes in different sizes, shapes, hair color, and eye color. So when you set goals, they should be yours and yours alone.

A few years ago I was training two women together who were close friends. These ladies have entirely different body types. Therefore, they had entirely different goals. One is five feet five inches tall and had been stuck at 155 pounds for about a year. She wanted to become more fit and lose 10 pounds. The other woman is five feet ten inches tall and weighed more than 200 pounds. Her goal was to lose 30 to 40 pounds and to reduce fat and build muscle.

At the beginning of our fitness program, it was clear that one of the women would quickly look better than the other. That's because one was more overweight than the other. I had to keep reminding the woman who needed to lose more weight to stay focused on herself and her personal goals. She couldn't compare herself to anyone else.

As I worked with my two friends, I realized that not everyone wants the same thing. Each person's goals are different, and they *should* be. A lot of women who set a goal to lose weight don't do it so they can fit into a size 6 or 8, especially if they start out as a size 16 or 18. Goals should be ambitious and challenging but realistic and doable.

The taller woman lost about 30 pounds in the first year. She started wearing a size 12 or 14. I began to think that with a bit more commitment and hard work, she could lose the additional 10 pounds she had talked about in the beginning. One day I said to her, "Are you ready to bring it home or what?" She looked at me, puzzled. Then she realized I was implying that she should lose the rest of what I considered to be her excess weight. She looked hurt and said to me quietly, "I bring it home every time I work out with you and every time I pass up the cheesecake after dinner at my favorite restaurant."

Ouch. I felt like such a jerk. She had come a *long* way, but I had the idea that she needed to keep going. The truth was she had already attained a healthy weight range and had maintained it for several months. She wasn't a perfect size 10, but she was making progress every day.

Every person has to determine the shape of the life she dreams about. You first decide to change your life, you reach the point of no return, and you commit to doing whatever it takes to live differently. You've desired a new life for some time. Now it's time to set a goal that is personal to you. You're the only one who can define the goals that will deliver the life you want.

DEATH TO PERFECTIONISM

With the One-Day Way, you're going to throw perfectionism out the window. I might picture you a year from now wearing a size 12, but the picture in my mind isn't what counts. Your ideal weight and dress size has to fit your vision for your life. Don't trust an article in a fashion magazine, don't be swayed by the Photoshopped pictures in magazines, and don't let your best friend or someone at the fitness center determine your goals. Your goals are yours alone.

Think of what you've done already. You tore down old habits that were working against you. You got rid of the temptation to compare yourself with others and to measure your success using an outside yardstick. Your new life is now under construction. You're rehabbing yourself to keep what you value in your life as you build in new aspects that you've been dreaming about for a long time.

In an earlier chapter we talked about avoiding self-defeating goals, such as focusing on a six-month outcome or an unrealistic weight-loss goal. I'm a life coach and a personal trainer, so I will never tell you that staying overweight is an option. You need to set a goal that will push you and challenge you to be the best you can be. At the same time, your goal must be personal to you. The woman I mentioned at the beginning of this chapter lost thirty pounds and attained a healthy weight. There's a wide range of what's healthy, and you have to do what works for you.

You might think I'm advocating an unhealthy emphasis on self. Perhaps you feel that focusing too much on your own needs and desires is wrong. You know the importance of serving others and sacrificing your own wants for the good of others. I hold those same values.

However, if you're committed to changing your life, you have to concentrate on yourself. If you don't invest effort in planning and goal setting, you won't be able to rebuild your life. Think about your bank account. If you fail to make regular deposits but continue to withdraw funds, eventually your account will be overdrawn. Trust me, this is very costly. Likewise, without making investments in yourself, which includes taking time each day to care for your body and your mind, you will have insufficient resources available. You'll lack the wherewithal to achieve your dreams.

Have you ever watched the television program *The Biggest Loser*? In each season premiere, the contestants look like they haven't paid attention to their personal appearance for years. It's as if the show's producers want to make the contestants look and feel pathetic, perhaps in an effort to fortify their desire to change. I think they may even deny the women access to lipstick. Sure, I get the reasoning behind making these people look hopeless. When you begin the series with contestants who look like they're knocking on death's door, it enhances the dramatic change from before to after.

When people need to change, sure, they have to have motivation and confidence to make it happen. But if you're trying to change because you feel pathetic, you won't be inspired over the long haul to give it everything you've got. And that's a problem. In the case of the people on *The Biggest Loser,* experts keep pressuring them to lose weight. But in real life, you're on your own. And after the cameras stop rolling, so are those contestants.

So start from a place of strength. You want to hold on to the things you value about your current life, and you've made a commitment to change the things that hold you back. Even though you are about to build a new life, you are far from pathetic. As you lay the foundation, think about your "before" photo. Mark on your calendar the day that you will wake up and begin your One-Day Way program. Then prepare yourself the night before. Set aside time to be alone with your thoughts. Have a notepad nearby to jot down ideas that come to you, and keep your camera handy. Turn on your favorite music, light your best-smelling candle, and fix yourself up. Comb your hair, and put on makeup and a nice outfit. Do whatever makes you feel the very best. Prepare as if you were going out to a nice restaurant. I know this sounds unconventional, but as you may have noticed by this point, I am a bit unconventional.

Make your "before" photo look great!

Here's why. The night I sat in my car in tears and finally admitted that I had to change once and for all, I was totally miserable. But I decided to begin to live with a new mission: I would be the best I could be each day. What pulled me out of my pain and gave me the power and strength to continue to press on was this: a love for myself and a desire to live better. Displaying an old photograph of me weighing nearly 350 pounds would have been a reminder of what I was escaping but not a motivation to seek a new life. Certainly it was not a cause for any kind of celebration.

I realized the woman I was in the car that night was *not* a flop and a failure. I was worth something! I was worth the investment of careful thought, planning, and focused effort. I could *do something* about my problem because I possessed serious value, not because I was pathetic. I was someone to be celebrated even in that moment of desperation. In fact, feeling that I was pathetic led mostly to negative self-talk, which had done nothing except keep me depressed.

When you're preparing to lay the foundation for your new life, envision the woman you want to become. You seek a new life, and you're willing to do the work required to lay hold of that life. So as you begin, value and appreciate the woman God has made you at this moment, whether you need to lose twenty pounds or a hundred.

The person you are right now, before any changes begin, is amazing and beautiful, worthwhile, special. You are a unique individual who will build a new life—one you have dreamed about but never knew how to achieve.

Getting Your Plan on Paper

When you begin to build your new life, the first thing to change is your thinking. You're going to overhaul your old mentality so you can change the way you think from now on. For example, you'll stop thinking in terms of dieting for the next six or twelve months. You won't put your hopes on losing a certain number of pounds by Christmas or summer break or this time next year. In fact, you'll let go of all time frames beyond the next twenty-four hours. There's a good reason for this. Too often your best efforts get sabotaged by worries about the future. If it's June and you're already worrying about how you're going to eat throughout the holidays, stop! Focus just on today. I'm telling you the truth. Obsessing over the future will prevent you from achieving the life you want to build.

So as you approach this new life one day at a time, figure out what you want to build. What kind of life are you constructing? Before a foundation is laid, an architect first has a vision and a perspective of what he's going to draw. Then he gets the specifics down on paper. He also has to know the foundation he needs to build on. Taking all of this into account will deliver the best possible results and ensure that the structure has beauty and ongoing usefulness.

Remember that the night before you begin the One-Day Way, you have fixed yourself up, you are dressed well, you have created a warm environment, and you are feeling good. Take out your notepad, because it's time to play architect. Draw a vertical line down the middle of a page. Write "What I love about me" across the top of one column and "What I'd love to change about me" at the top of the other. And then fire away. The only rule is that for each item you list on one side, there must be a corresponding item on the other side.

If you have something you want to change about your appearance, then write something in the other column that you *like* about your appearance. If you write down something you really like about your personality or your inner self, be sure to match it with something you'd love to change about your attitude. For instance, if in one column you write that you like being a generous person, in the other column note perhaps that you want to start being more generous with yourself.

When you list your goal to lose weight, write in the other column something you love about your appearance. If you love the fact that you're a great cook, you might put on the other side "I'd love to cook healthier meals during the week." The list is entirely yours, so make it as long as you want. A long list simply means you are serious about reconstructing your body and your life.

Don't overlook the positive ways you influence others. Include things like "I love that I am a great friend" or "I'd love to deliver a meal once a month to an elderly person." Remember, part of who you are is reflected in your willingness to serve others. After your list is complete, put it in a place where you'll see it every day. Then do a few touch-ups to your makeup and hair, crank up the music, hold your camera at arm's length from your face, smile big, and click! You are a confident, eager, committed person who is about to start building a new body and a new life. Try to capture who you are today, even though you're in for some major changes. This day, this one special and monumental day, is the start of something significant. It's the day you finally decided to believe you're worth it. And it's the day you've chosen to commit to becoming the best you can be without worrying about the distant future—while letting go of the past.

Print the picture and put it with your list, perhaps in your bathroom taped to the mirror or in the kitchen stuck on the fridge. When you walk by and see the photo, focus on something you love about yourself. I know this can be difficult, because most people feel weird saying something positive about themselves. But in reality, when you do this, you're complimenting your Creator.

After all, He's the One who selected just the right height, hair color, and eye color for you. You had nothing to do with these traits. But acknowledging them is a great way to recognize something positive that you possess today.

Reconstructing yourself is an exciting process. But be aware that if you're not careful, others can distract you from your project. At times you may need to stay away from someone who could bring you down or divert you. (If it's your spouse, don't tell him I said you should sleep in the next room!) I'm talking more about influences outside your home. Just as a recovering alcoholic stays away from his drinking buddies, you may have to keep a healthy distance from relationships that could be toxic to your efforts to change.

One simple strategy when you're initially trying to lose weight is to avoid frequent meetings and social engagements that involve eating. I encourage you to schedule hang-out time with others based on sharing conversation instead of a dessert or a pizza. For example, meet at a park or the library. Look out for yourself. It's your life you're building, so do what it takes to get it right. You may even need to consider putting some relationships on hold for a season.

A few years ago I was part of a group of girlfriends who had dinner together once a month. We called it "girls' night out," but it should have been called "mommies' complaintfest." It wasn't the food that troubled me; it was the conversation. Each time we gathered, the evening was spent complaining about our children, our husbands, or our physical imperfections. I value relationships that involve being real, but there was never any edification in the exchanges. None of us left feeling built up or encouraged. There is enough in the world that tears us down, so avoid situations like this one whenever possible.

You're the architect on this building project, and the project is *you*! The One-Day Way is a lifestyle built on the foundation of a new way of thinking. Instead of worrying about big goals, you must take small, doable steps. We're working toward progress, not perfection.

. . . .

Chapter 7

It's All About Progress, Not Perfection

Bite-Size Successes Bring You Further Along

I recently spent an afternoon with Susan (not her real name). I had sent her some signed copies of my books at the request of a close friend of mine, who was Susan's friend.

Susan and I shared a few tears as she described her past attempts to lose weight. She had tried numerous diets and fitness programs, but she hadn't been able to stick with them. She now needed to lose at least 175 pounds to get within a healthy weight range. As I listened to her story, I realized the recurring theme was fear. Susan was afraid to try my fitness program because she believed she wouldn't be able to stay on it. She was afraid of making mistakes, and she dreaded the thought that she might be set-ting herself up for yet another failure. As often happens when people are ruled by fear, she had an all-or-nothing mind-set. She thought that if she took small steps, it wouldn't be enough.

Whether you need to lose 175 pounds or 17, you still lose it a pound at a time. It's easy to be overwhelmed by the enormity of the task. We feel we have too many bad habits to break, too many pounds to lose, too many past failures to overcome. Susan told me about her nightly ritual of eating a bowl (or two) of ice cream. She knew it was an unhealthy habit, and she realized it wasn't the only destructive habit that held her back. She needed to trust the power of tak-ing small steps.

I explained the freeing approach in the One-Day Way. I told Susan that just giving up ice cream for a day would empower her. That small step, which anyone could do, would boost her confidence and build her sense of taking control of her life. Initially, she had trouble accepting my advice. She truly believed that unless she gave up *everything* in an instant—all the unhealthy food she enjoyed, all the sedentary habits of her life—she'd always be stuck needing to lose 175 pounds.

It's never easy to lose weight, and I agreed with Susan that she had a big task ahead of her. But if she allowed fear to keep her from taking the first step, she would keep feeling like a failure. She needed to change the way she was thinking so she could then change her life. Believing that she had to give up everything at once kept her stuck in a life she didn't want.

I explained the concept of bite-size success. If she could taste a few victo-ries, even small ones, she would be able to build from there. Because she admit-ted that a nightly bowl or two of ice cream was something she could change, I told her to start there. Could she forgo the ice cream for one day? Then could she repeat the same success by deciding to skip it again the next day? That would be a great start: to do one thing for one day. And the next day to do it again.

I had her add a simple, thirty-minute cardio session every day. Now, for someone who is nearly 200 pounds overweight, doing thirty minutes of cardio every day is a huge change. But it's just one thing, and it's a change that can be made in one day. If she could do that and taste bite-size success, it would inspire her to make further changes on other days.

THINK DIFFERENTLY, ACT DIFFERENTLY

Talking about changes is a good start, but for it to have a lasting effect, you have to make a commitment to act on your new thinking. I pulled out the Brain Change Contract from my book *Never Say Diet* for Susan to sign and for me to witness. This contract is similar to the One-Day Way Contract you'll see in chapter 16. It's an agreement to help you stay on track, to hold you accountable to the changes you're making.

I asked Susan to read the words out loud, stating the commitments with all the conviction she could muster. Just as she began to read the contract, one of the arms of the chair she was sitting in snapped, and she began to fall. I was so embarrassed for her, but she didn't seem too upset. In fact, she smiled sheepishly and brushed off the incident, saying, "Well, that's not the first time that's happened."

I looked at her and said, "But if you want it to be the last, it can be. You don't have to experience that feeling again, ever." I then set up an agreement with her involving a personal accountability system. In one week I would expect to receive a text message about something worth celebrating. Susan would have found one thing each day to move her closer to healthier living. Also, she had to update me with reports that she had moved enough to break a sweat for a half hour every day. That would show she was committed to daily cardio exercise.

To my delight, on Sunday afternoon the words "…and on the seventh day she rested" appeared on my phone. I wanted to shout hallelujah! Susan was on course. She had tasted small successes each day that week, and it showed. I knew from experience that the joy and excitement of feeling this good had the power to carry her through to the next week. Not because she weighed in and saw a big difference. More importantly, because she had made a commitment and had kept her promise to herself. As I wrote this chapter, I received another Sunday text. Susan is living the One-Day Way and getting healthier, stronger, and more confident all the time!

In the previous chapter we talked about your being the architect of your new life. You made a list of things you love about yourself and things you want to change. But how do you make that change happen? You succeed in big changes by doing things one piece at a time. No renovation happens overnight. You reach success by continually tasting it, taking a small bite every day.

In this chapter I'll give you practical steps you can take to live the One-Day Way one day at a time. Instead of thinking about the food you don't get to eat, focus on taking a bite of success. Every day you can taste the feeling of accomplishment—if you choose to. When I was losing weight, I made sure every day to do something that would challenge me. In fact, I still do this, because the One-Day Way is not a short-term program; it's a lifestyle. One day I might challenge myself to walk at the highest incline setting on the treadmill that I could tolerate for five minutes. Another day my challenge might be to go online to discover a new healthy chicken recipe that my family would enjoy. Each day something new, something gratifying. It's that simple.

This is where you have to get creative and figure out your own daily challenge. While I will give you help and encouragement (there are suggestions at the end of this chapter), your success is ultimately up to you! Believe that you can do this! You're more creative than you think you are, and trusting yourself is part of the foundation necessary for reconstruction. It's your life, your dreams, your goals, and your desire to change. You will make it happen.

Our son Jake has become an avid reader. I laugh sometimes because, truthfully, my husband and I could never have taught him this. Even though I'm an author, I'm not the "book pusher" type. However, it's exciting to always find my son immersed in a new adventure. It has gotten to the point where I've found him taking a shower with his book propped open next to him. (Since he's nine years old, if the shower is more than three minutes, I'm thrilled.)

Recently Jake began setting a personal goal each day. He'd decide at breakfast how many pages he would get through that day. He would flip ahead in the book, look for an interesting place to stop, and make that number of pages his goal. I don't need to tell you what has happened as a result of his little system. At bedtime he's often furiously cramming in those last few pages so he can meet his goal. Which is awesome and exciting! I love what he's doing with reading, because it's exactly what I've done in living a healthy lifestyle. He loves to read, so he sets a goal for one day. That's the same way we change our life. Every morning we have a new day, we set a goal, and we change our life one day at a time.

The Sweet Taste of Success

What are some things you can begin to do to taste success on a regular basis? What small steps can you take? These things can be related to any of the three key construction materials: faith, food, or fitness. Some days you can taste success that involves all three. Every morning think about at least one thing in one area you'll be sure to do. Whatever you choose, it's a commitment you make to yourself. And it's for that day.

Say, for example, you have a habit of eating two oatmeal-raisin cookies every afternoon when you get home from work. Your challenge might be to skip the cookies for a day. When you get home from work that day, instead of staring at the cookie jar, take a walk around the block. That's actually two changes, but they're connected. The brisk walk will distract you from thinking about cookies! Your success is based on progress toward breaking negative habits and replacing them with constructive habits.

One of my favorite restaurants is Seasons 52, a chain that has a few locations in South Florida. This restaurant prides itself on serving dishes made with seasonal vegetables. They also have an awesome dessert concept. After the meal they bring over a tray with an amazing array of treats—all tantalizing in miniature glass containers. Seriously, there isn't much more than three good bites in each one. Which means they are all low calorie, regardless of how rich. Even the pecan pie contains less than three hundred calories when they slice it and serve it this way.

This whole thing is ingenious. First of all, the first bite or two always taste the best. This is true with any food—be it an appetizer, main course, or dessert. Once you get past the first few bites, most likely you keep eating because it's in front of you, not because you're savoring it. You're certainly not hungry. Second, having something, in moderation, that's really good preserves the integrity of food as a special treat, especially if you're having a bit of dessert. An amazing dessert should be a delight, not an add-on that makes you feel stuffed. (Is it a treat if it makes you grab an antacid at bedtime?)

So have a bite of food. Then stop. It's a small success; you still get to enjoy the delicious dessert, and you can build your confidence with this victory. What a sweet way to start changing your life. I'm talking not about just small bits of food but small steps toward improving your health and fitness.

So achieve your goals by doing things small! Each day give yourself a small but significant challenge, and accomplish it. Taste success, even in a small bite. These steps are filling but will still keep you wanting more. The fact that you've accomplished something, even if it is small, will help you stay the course on days when you would otherwise consider giving up. Today's small success will build you up so you can overcome a setback or frustration next week. Bite-size success is addictive! Use it to your personal benefit.

What Bite-Size Success Looks Like

To help you get started, here are some bite-size success ideas that you can sink your teeth into. These ideas all relate to food, one of the three tools we're using to build a new life. As you give these a try, keep in mind that you can come up with new ones. Your daily goal is to find a challenge small enough to reach for and achieve in a day, yet big enough to stretch you. Try any one of these for just one day. The next day try another. Then the next day be creative and try a personal challenge that you come up with on your own.

- Give up all snack foods (for example, granola bars, 100-calorie packs).
- Drink water only. (This means no coffee or diet soda either. Headache time!)
- Find a protein source other than meat, and eat that instead. (Be creative; tofu is terrific.)
- Have only fruit before noon. (Two bananas and two apples contain only 350 calories. Crazy, right?)
- Try to starve your sweet tooth by eating nothing with sugar, including fresh fruit. (It's important not to feed your sweet tooth all the time.)
- Have only veggies for snacks. (They crunch like potato chips but are healthy.)
- Stop eating after 5 p.m. (Make it an early dinner.)
- Don't eat anything prepared by anyone but you (even if your mama made it!).

- Choose to have protein at each meal, and eat it first. (You will feel full much more quickly.)
- Don't eat anything unless you're sitting down. (Slow down your eating as you take time to count your blessings.)

Doing something every day that is challenging will not only increase your fitness; it will build your faith. You will reap major rewards if you're mindful of the role faith plays in your life. Faith is defined as believing in something you can't see.[3] Making physical improvements, working on relationships, or seeing your future plans come to fruition requires faith, and it grows your faith. In other words, taking on tasks that cause you to be uncomfortable will help you grow. Here are ten One-Day Ways to challenge you in the area of faith:

1. Write a letter forgiving someone who has offended you (even if that person hasn't apologized).
2. Make a list of places you would like to travel to, and pick your top one. (Get it on your calendar.)
3. Ask your co-workers how you can help them get a task done. (If you're the supervisor, ask your employees.)
4. Tell ten people how much you appreciate them being in your life. (Twenty would be even better.)
5. It's "count your blessings day." Think of a new one at the top of every hour. (This is a piece of cake.)
6. Don't go near a computer or television after work. Instead, go for a family walk (all of you).
7. Buy a new pair of jeans that won't zip. (That's serious faith!)
8. Give twenty dollars to someone in need, and tell them to give five dollars of it away to someone else. (This is fun.)
9. Who annoys you the most? Send or give them a card, saying, "I'm thinking of you." (Not easy!)

10. Pick out an outfit you love from a catalog, and order it when you know it will fit. (Exciting!)

Here are bite-size successes in the area of fitness. Give them a try!

- Try a new form of cardio exercise for thirty minutes. (But don't go Rollerblading without proper protective gear.)
- Make the last five minutes of your workout extra intense. (You'll recover eventually.)
- Invite someone you love to sweat with you. (Just remember your Soft and Dry.)
- Don't eat within four hours prior to your workout. (You'll burn lots of fat. Is this okay with you?)
- Get up an hour earlier than usual, and go for a walk. (It makes for a great prayer time!)
- Hop on a treadmill, and increase the incline every three minutes for the session. (Go for it!)
- While doing your strength training, do jumping jacks between sets. (Good-bye, calories.)
- After a great workout, write down ten reasons you love to exercise. (Keep the list handy.)
- Put on your favorite music, and do sit-ups to every other song. (Find the rhythm.)
- Add fifteen minutes to your cardio workout, and during the extra minutes push yourself a little more every two minutes. (Be sure to give 100 percent.)

These lists are suggestions to get you going and help you take a bite out of success. They'll help you begin to lay the foundation for a whole new way of thinking and a whole new way of living. And more changes are in store. Next, we need to change the way we think about the screwups and setbacks in our lives.

Denise's One-Day Way Story

I honestly can't remember a time when I didn't struggle with my weight. My mother put me on a diet when I was eight, and from then on it seemed like I was constantly being reprimanded. I felt like people were judging me anytime I put something in my mouth. I heard, "You know you need to lose weight!" and, "You can't eat like other kids."

I decided to start eating in secret. I would binge on chips, cookies, candy, or chocolate—whatever I could get my hands on. I remember eating a whole watermelon once.

By the time I got to high school, I was one of the heaviest girls in my school. When I graduated, I stood at just over five feet tall and weighed 220 pounds. I used to cry myself to sleep, asking God to make me normal. I never understood why I had to be fat. I tried so many different diets, pills, shakes, even laxatives to lose weight. But nothing worked.

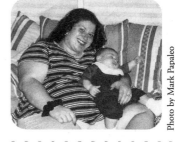

Photo by Mark Papaleo

I got married as an overweight bride and then had a near-death experience after giving birth. I was completely depressed about my weight. Then one day I realized I had a choice! I lost the extra weight from my pregnancy and dropped to 212 pounds. However, once I felt better, I stopped dieting and went back to my old binging style, eating my way to 270 pounds.

My emotions were as up and down as my weight, and things got worse. For the next four and a half years, I suffered from panic disorder, then severe depression. Despite medication, I was in a dark hole of fear, obsessed with sickness and fears of dying. My compulsions became worse. I was a complete hypochondriac.

When I had a miscarriage in 1999, I was sad but relieved because I was so afraid of getting sick again. But later I decided I was not going to let fear take any more of my life from me. With a lot of prayer and guidance, I planned my next pregnancy and decided to get my act together. I started watching what I ate. I was down to 208 pounds when I found out I was pregnant with my daughter. Throughout my pregnancy I became focused. My mission was to be the best I could be for my children.

I also learned how to control negative self-talk and behavior. I can honestly say I grew stronger than I imagined I could be. On September 3, 2002, before I gave birth to my beautiful baby Samantha, I weighed 188 pounds. I actually lost weight during my pregnancy simply by making better choices one day at a time.

After my daughter's birth, I found myself getting a little off track, and I gained about 10 pounds. I felt I was losing control again. But one day something simple changed my outlook. My cousin, whom I had always admired for her healthy, fit lifestyle, came to see the baby. I put coffeecake and fruit on the table. She chose to eat fruit and not cake. Something just clicked: I saw her make a better choice. I was never the same again.

Six months later I became pregnant with my third child, Sophia. I was down to 156 pounds, and better yet, I was exercising. While I was pregnant, I would put Samantha in her bouncy seat, put on some music for me and a Barney tape for her, and walk for thirty minutes on a treadmill.

The thing that supported the outward changes was an inner change: I no longer worried about the future but tried to cultivate a day-to-day, "let go and let God" attitude. I was trusting God and living without fear.

Photo by Mark Papaleo

It was around this time when I met Chantel Hobbs, who taught Spinning at my gym. I decided to take her class even though I was a bit scared. I was amazed at how inspiring and motivating she was. The energy in that room was incredible. Soon after meeting Chantel, I told her my story. From then on she was my mentor. She helped me through every Spin class. It felt like God had sent her to me.

I decided I also wanted to inspire and motivate people to be their best one day at a time, one workout at a time. This was the message I had heard in Chantel's class. Working hard one day at a time was how I had achieved my own goals. Soon I started teaching Spinning and took over one of Chantel's classes.

How can we take care of the people and things in our lives that we love if we don't first take care of ourselves? You have to live with this thought: today is here; make it count.

When I weighed 280 pounds and would think about how much weight I had to lose, it overwhelmed me. My goal of achieving a healthy weight was so far away! But once I started taking it one day at a time, enjoying the journey, I got closer and closer to my goals.

Chapter 8

. . . .

A Better Way to Think About Accidents, Screwups, and Setbacks

Turn the Past into a Positive Force

o you remember a commercial from the 1970s that introduced us to Reese's Peanut Butter Cups? It opened with a guy walking down the street, eating peanut butter straight out of the jar. Coming around the corner was a woman holding her cat and eating a chocolate bar. Because both people were enjoying themselves so much, they weren't watching where they were going. They collided, snacks first. "You put chocolate in my peanut butter," he says. "And you put peanut butter in my chocolate," she exclaims. And there you have it, folks, the yummy delight and perfect PMS cure: the peanut butter cup!

Now ask yourself: was this collision the scene of an accident, a screwup, a setback, or simply serendipity? I prefer to think of it as serendipitous. It wasn't planned, but look at the positive outcome. Peanut butter and chocolate—what a combination!

We've all done things in the past that we regret. We've attempted things and failed. We've given up on achieving goals rather than sticking with our plan. We've given in to bad habits and felt guilty about it later. But all of that is in the past, and this is today. The past is behind us for one good reason—it's done. There is nothing we can do today that will change yesterday or last year.

A New Look at the Past

Starting today, when certain events from the past come to mind, focus on what you learned from those experiences—good or bad. If you're troubled by a past failure to stick with a fitness program, consider the things you learned about what prevented you from following through. If you had success losing weight and then, over time, regained it, think about the forces that influenced you to go back to your old ways.

You have the power to choose to see the things from your past, including the setbacks, in a positive light. Understanding that things happen for a reason and finding the silver lining of every gray cloud that looms will set you free. Instead of being tormented by old hurts and disappointments, you'll be able to see how the struggles taught you valuable lessons and eventually inspired you to change. The past has the power to propel you into a new life rather than holding you back.

Accidents

An accident is something that just happens, right? It can't be planned for, and it can't be foreseen. You may be going about your business one day, following your normal routine, when something happens, and then the whole world feels as if it has been turned upside down.

Screwups

A screwup, on the other hand, is the label we put on a poor choice or a mistake. Someone is at fault and has made a mistake that has consequences for others. You've been affected at times by others' actions that you had no control over. At other times you were responsible for the screwup. You knew what the right thing was, but you chose to do the wrong thing.

Setbacks

Accidents and screwups often result in setbacks. A setback delays our progress. It introduces a detour we didn't expect. But does that have to be the case? Do screwups always have to become setbacks? What if we were able to see the good in an apparent setback? What if we had a different mind-set, one that led us to think differently about accidents, screwups, and setbacks? Remember the accidental collision of peanut butter and chocolate. It wasn't a setback at all but a serendipity!

Serendipity

Serendipity leads to surprises and delightful outcomes. Serendipity is finding the value in things we didn't plan for, didn't seek out, and didn't want to happen. What if we could learn to look at our accidents as opportunities? see our screwups as starting points? view seeming setbacks as success builders? We'd be living serendipitous lives every day and making progress as a result. This means each time we set out to accomplish a goal, we'd realize that everything that happens, even what appears to be a step backward, is bringing us closer to some measure of achievement! Serendipitous thinking keeps you in the moment, concentrating on your life today and freeing you from the bonds of the past.

It's not easy to think this way. Several years ago when I was in the middle of my weight loss, I had what I thought was a setback. It took me awhile to realize that it was a serendipitous blessing. Here's what happened.

My husband, Keith, our kids, and I were on our way home from our annual fall trip to the Great Smoky Mountains. As we got closer to home, I began to feel sick. I knew this form of nausea well—I had felt it a few times years earlier. As our Suburban pulled into the driveway, I dragged myself out of the car and crawled straight to bed.

The next morning I drove to the store, still feeling shocked and in denial, and picked up a home pregnancy test. As soon as I got home, I headed straight to the bathroom. With my hands shaking and my mind fearing "the worst," I waited what seemed like two eternal minutes. This silly piece of plastic possessed the ability to predict the next year of my life, and that made me angry. You see, I had already lost 180 pounds. I loved my children, but a pregnancy would really mess up my plan to continue to lose weight and to enjoy the smaller jeans I was fitting into.

My suspicions were confirmed as I took a deep breath and looked down. Nothing about this was going to be easy! Through tear-filled eyes I was definitely seeing two purple lines. *How could this have happened?* While I thought I knew biology, my body had decided not to follow the rules.

The next few weeks were a blur of exhaustion and sleepless nights filled with countless mind games. Whenever I recalled conversations I'd had with women who couldn't get pregnant or who had suffered a miscarriage, I'd feel awful that I'd been complaining about being pregnant. But that didn't keep me from feeling awful about being pregnant.

I had finally tasted success in losing weight. Now I'd have to put my self-improvement program on hold for several months. I was mad about how the impending arrival of new life would affect the new life I'd been working so hard to achieve. I had to find a way to move forward, one day at a time. One wasted meal I would order and then be too nauseated to eat—at a time. One newly fitting pair of jeans that had to be hidden away—at a time.

It was useless to look backward, because I couldn't change the past. But today, many years after the birth of my youngest child, I look back and see something beautiful. I see now that my pregnancy with Luke was not an accident or a screwup but a serendipitous event.

First of all, it showed me I'd been taking too much credit for the work I felt I'd done. The truth is, I hadn't done all the work. God's strength coupled with my commitment had gotten me to the point of losing so much weight. I also realized that the accomplishment hadn't ended just because my body was going to change for a period of time. Once I refocused on my mission to be the best I could be every day, my pregnancy was filled with great joy. My faith and confidence grew in a way they never had before as the months progressed.

You see, friend, becoming the best I can be is going to be a personal challenge for as long as I live. Even when I was handling the emotions of pregnancy, the mission was the same. My physical state changed for several months, but that was only temporary. Once I realized that, I made being the best pregnant woman I could be my top priority. That change in thinking taught me a great lesson that I still use all the time. I will never be off the hook. I've grown stronger against allowing excuses to overpower my desire to stay fit, strong, and healthy. And don't get me wrong. Sometimes the excuses are valid, such as a lack of energy, morning sickness, a packed schedule. No matter what, I will stay the course.

SETBACK OR SERENDIPITY?

Each week of my pregnancy, I grew more and more excited to meet this child I had learned so much from. But one day about a month before he was due, as I walked around a store looking for baby furniture, I felt a sharp and unfamiliar pain. I grabbed Keith's arm and begged him to take me straight to the hospital. I'd had three children before, and I knew something was not right. Later that night the Hobbs family welcomed Luke Allen via an emergency cesarean. Because his lungs were full of fluid, he was rushed away from me and taken to intensive care. I didn't even have the opportunity to see his face.

There I lay on a cold table, stretched out on what looked like a cross, having my vital signs monitored constantly. I was scared, shivering. Even as my body was sewn back together from a near uterine rupture, my heart was ripping apart. I felt sick, empty. I desperately missed the little life that had been growing for all those months in my womb. I just prayed, "God, help me, help my baby fight."

In the midst of the darkness and fear, I heard God speak to my heart: *Trust Me, daughter. I was the One who wiped your teary eyes over this pregnancy, washed them with hope, and replaced them with overwhelming excitement. Let go. He was My son before I gifted him to you.* I had no idea that several years afterward I would come to a place where I would need to hear, remember, and cling to those words.

Truthfully, those hours were some of the longest of my life. When Luke came home to join the rest of the family, I felt more alive and complete than ever before. The events of the previous nine months were all part of the mosaic of my life and my transformation. Losing the baby weight and regaining my fitness level wasn't as hard as I'd feared. I was able to refocus even though there were still challenges ahead.

THE PHONE CALL EVERYONE FEARS

Two years later my trust in God was tested again when I got the worst phone call I've ever received. When I heard the voice on the line say, "Are you Keith's wife?" I quickly said I was, but all I could think was, *This can't be happening.* In the background I could hear sirens and lots of noise. The man on the phone informed me that my husband and sons had been involved in a roll-over accident. He said he had no further information. "Just get to Broward trauma center, and hurry."

I was already in the car and immediately started the thirty-minute drive to the hospital. I was met by television cameras, but there was no one I loved in sight. Within a few minutes they arrived. A Life Flight helicopter brought my son Jake, who was five at the time. Then Luke and finally Keith. Their eyes were open, and I desperately longed to hold each one to comfort him. As much as I begged, I couldn't go to any of them. Something about internal injuries. Finally, hours later, I was able to hug and touch each one.

I found out that the reporters were there because the accident had been caused by teenagers who were drag racing, dodging in and out of traffic, on the road that my family was traveling on. I was told later by an investigator that, upon impact, our truck had flipped seven times. Luke was ejected as this nearly six-thousand-pound vehicle tumbled over and over. No one could prevent the seat belt from breaking away from his car seat. All the faith and planning couldn't have stopped this accident from taking place. No preparation on my part could have made these young men decide not to endanger others with their reckless driving.

But in a serendipitous world, I still get to sing my son to sleep, thankful again and again that he entered my life. I know the tears I shed over that pregnancy test prepared me for the most desperate prayers I would ever pray, waiting in a hospital corridor. And God answered my prayers within a few days. Without one stitch being necessary or any bones needing to be set, Keith, Jake, and Luke were released to come home.

The Past Is a Foundation

Here's what I know: to build a solid foundation for your new life, you need to see life's events as pieces that fit together to produce something worthwhile. Don't get stuck in guilt or regret or blame. Choose to be extraordinary, and learn how to see each day's trials and disappointments as serendipity instead of setbacks.

One of my favorite places to visit in New York City is a little restaurant on the Upper East Side called Serendipity. I first saw it featured on *Oprah* years ago. The spot is famous for serving frozen hot chocolate. It sounds weird—frozen hot chocolate? But I'm telling you, when you taste it, it just works! It is utterly delicious.

So many things about my life are frozen hot chocolate. They don't make sense. So many times I've felt that I couldn't make it another day, that I'm the only one who could be feeling this much pain. But what I'm learning, even now, is that we all can grow stronger and be better if we'll let go of trying to make sense of everything. The past has a purpose. It led to you becoming the person you are today. It's up to you to choose how to view what happened in the past. Accidents, setbacks, failures, or serendipity? Those who dreamed up peanut butter cups and frozen hot chocolate know the answer.

. . . .

Chapter 9

How to Throw a Private Party

Celebrating Your Success Is What Matters

In years past I loved throwing huge parties for lots of people. The more, the merrier; no invitation needed; come one, come all. I found that whenever free food and karaoke were involved, everyone would show up— and so would their relatives. If fewer than fifty people came to one of my extravaganzas, I felt like the event was a flop.

Looking back, I can see this was crazy on so many levels. First of all, the larger the group, the more work I had to do to get ready. Second, regardless of the number of people who showed up, I felt pressure to spend time with all of them. Because this was impossible, inevitably I would be mad at myself when I said good-bye to someone and realized I hadn't talked to that person earlier. Finally, by the time the night was over, I felt drained. It was as if the life had been sucked out of me.

So why put myself through this? That's what I would ask after beating myself upside the head too many times to count. Why did I continue to plan these events if I never fully enjoyed them?

Now that I'm a recovered "party-throwing queen," I'll tell you. It boils down to the need to feel validated. I was desperate to have everyone I knew come to my house and tell me I was a really good cook and I had a lovely home. I couldn't wait for them to top it off by asking, "How do you get it all done?" Pretty sad and pathetic, I know. By the time my last guest would leave, I'd be frazzled.

Maybe you aren't the type to throw huge parties. But I'd bet you find other ways to try to earn approval—your own method for getting people to validate you. And while we all need encouragement, sometimes we go too far in trying to make other people happy. In an effort to win approval, we sacrifice ourselves and our sanity.

Stop Trying to Earn Approval

If you see yourself in this story, it might shed some light on your struggles with your weight. The plain truth is that we don't need other people to validate us. God has already done that. You are valuable not because anyone praises your cooking or your abilities as a hostess but because God made you. The realization that others don't determine my worth led me to throw my first private party. I call it a private party because it was by invitation only, it was limited, and it was designed for everyone—me included—to fully enjoy the evening.

As I planned this small party, I looked forward to spending quality time with a small group of people. I invited four special couples that we enjoy being with but who didn't know one another before that evening.

Rather than serving a complicated menu, I kept things simple and was able to prepare a lot the day before the party. I found myself looking forward to this gathering more than any party I'd ever planned. I focused on details that made it more personal and special. Because I had only eight guests, I created an intimate table setting and placed name cards to welcome each person to his or her spot. Since I didn't have to buy massive quantities of food, I could focus on quality and plan a gourmet menu. With fewer things to do in advance, I used the extra time to make a disc of relaxing music to play in the background.

The party was a delight. Each couple arrived hand in hand with a smile on their faces, and because the group was small, I was able to greet them and make introductions. After we savored the appetizers, the evening progressed to a three-hour dinner by candlelight. The conversations were meaningful, and I can honestly say I didn't want the evening to end. Later we gathered in my kitchen, and I whipped up some Bananas Foster. I lit the flame on the dessert and served my special friends with pure joy. My private party was personal and relaxed. I was delighted with the thought-provoking and encouraging conversation. And I loved connecting these friends to each other. I threw a great small party, and I felt free. I didn't throw a party so I could feel better about myself. I hosted a party for enjoyment and to connect people I cared about.

THROW YOUR OWN PARTY

As you personalize the One-Day Way program, keep in mind that private parties are the perfect celebrations. You may think that in order to succeed in changing your life, you'll need a crowd around to cheer you on. You might assume you'll be relying on the support of a lot of people. And secretly you may be looking for approval from others. But I want you to think of this as your own private party. It's your life that you're building, and your choices and actions will make it happen. You can't make anyone else happy; you can only pursue your own dreams and achieve your own goals. When you can let go of trying to please everyone, you'll begin to find freedom and enjoyment in life.

It's true you will need support, but that should come from a select few. Decide now that you will let into your life only those people who are life giving and life affirming. Look objectively at the people you spend time with. Do they seem to take from you but never give anything back? Then you need to take them off your guest list. No longer will you need them for validation. The primary thing to focus on is one small, bite-size success, one day at a time, with the support of a few close friends. You need friends who will affirm you as you reconstruct your life, friends who won't feel threatened by your success.

With your One-Day Way of living, you will enjoy the freedom to be more selective about who is included in your support system. And with fewer people involved, you'll be able to invest time in these people. These few relationships will go deeper, because you won't be trying to give to everyone you've ever met.

I know people who started a weight-loss program, and as soon as a friend said, "Oh, I tried that program, and it didn't work," they gave up! Why? Because they allowed other people to make choices for them. Especially when people are negative, you don't have to listen to them. Stay away from toxic people.

Sometimes we worry about letting people down. Remember my friend Susan from chapter 7? Even as she signed the contract, sitting in her broken chair, she was scared. What if she failed and let me down? I had to tell her very firmly, "If you fail, that is not going to mess me up. I will still be a marathon runner. I will still be living a healthy life. I'm hoping and praying you'll succeed, but you aren't doing this for me or anyone else. You have to do it for *you*." I wasn't being heartless; I was being helpful. You see, the only way to have personal change is to take personal responsibility. Your decisions, your success or failure won't help or harm someone else. It will help or harm you. You're reconstructing your own life; your choices will affect you. Others have to make their own choices.

Sometimes it's hard to find people who are positive and encouraging. One way to find positive people is to *become* a positive person. Find ways to be the encourager you want others to be for you. This doesn't mean letting them manipulate you in order to get them to like you. Rather, it means that you work to become a positive influence on others. Perhaps you wish others would be kind to you or would encourage you. Don't wait for them to go first. Treat them as you'd like to be treated. Become a person who encourages others.

Letting go of trying to make others happy allows your relationships to become healthier. You'll feel recharged and blessed after spending time with a smaller group of supporters, a private party of people who are on your side.

Now, there will be times when the only one at your private party is you. And that's okay. Because don't forget, the One-Day Way is personal. You don't have to waste your energy trying to get other people to jump onto your bandwagon. It's nice to do the One-Day Way program with a friend or your spouse, but you don't have to. It can be just you, celebrating your small steps of success.

DON'T SKIP THE PRIVATE CELEBRATIONS

Each time you pull off a bite-size success, such as tackling your first Spinning class, adding a second thirty-minute walk to your day, ordering only coffee at the drive-through, skipping the doughnut on the way to the office, or letting your child eat his chicken nuggets without your help, you'll feel energized. Celebrate your success! You chose the better option, and you followed through. Don't let your definition of success be based on other people's standards.

Private celebrations are best because they come from your private desires. Whatever you want to accomplish is within your reach as long as it's based on committing each day to doing the things you need to do. You also get to choose the ones you want to take along with you. When you handpick the people you will be close to and what you will accomplish and celebrate each day, blessings begin to flow.

The One-Day Way of living will ultimately give you the best parties you've ever had.

. . . .

PART 3

Building the Structure— a New You

Where to Find the Materials, Energy, and Labor for the Project

. . . .

Chapter 10

How to Turn On the Switch

The One-Day Way Faith Focus Is Your Electricity

I probably should have known that shopping at Hollister, the hip, trendy, surfer-style shop at the mall, was risky. But my daughters and I were walking past the store when we saw a brown shirt that we thought Keith might like. (Okay, I realized that the shirt might have been a bit tighter than he usually wears. Plus, just seeing a shopping bag from this store would definitely raise his right eyebrow.)

When I got home and excitedly pulled the shirt out of the bag, it wasn't the style or the store it came from that made Keith's eyes pop open. It was the color—purple!

Even Ashley and Kayla believed we had seen a brown shirt in the store display. But it was definitely purple and definitely not something Keith would wear.

So I had to return it—a chore I really, really dislike. Even if I bring the receipt, I still have to plop down my driver's license and hand over the credit card. If I'm standing there with a few of my offspring in tow, why would anyone need to know anything else about me? I'm Chantel Hobbs, not a terrorist masquerading as a Florida mom. Yet for some reason, the person processing the return always asks for more: e-mail address, phone number… *What's next,* I've wondered. *A blood sample, a saliva swab?* It's all so aggravating, which is exactly what they're going for. They want shoppers to give careful consideration before they dare return an item. And believe me, now I do.

But I had to return the shirt. After waiting in line, then waiting even longer for a manager, I finally got to hand over the purple apparel. Or at least I got a chance to try. The manager wanted to know the reason for the return.

I told him quite seriously that the reason for my return was a lack of light! "Your store is too dark," I explained. "I didn't get a good look at what I thought I was buying." It's challenging enough to find clothes that fit and for a good price. But now it seems some of the stores at the mall are so concerned with creating a party atmosphere or hip ambiance that the lights are dimmed. Is this a commercial enterprise or a middle-school make-out session? It's funny—not being able to actually see what you're buying can lead to a returned item.

WE ALL NEED BETTER VISION

We often make mistakes simply because we can't see clearly. Yet with a little more power and more light, we would make better decisions, because we would have more information. Every decision we make hinges on what we can and can't see. We're limited, so we can't see everything. And that's why we need faith. Faith is believing in what we can't see.[4] It is the backbone of the choices we make, the actions we take, and the challenges we'll choose.

It takes faith to believe you can make a commitment and stick to it. Sure, you're the one making the choices and taking the necessary actions, every day, to make good on a commitment. But we all know we can be weak, and we tend to second-guess our decisions. Faith adds another dimension that can carry us through the times when we want to give up and go back to the old life we're trying to escape.

As we've seen, the One-Day Way has three essential building materials: faith, food, and fitness. These three elements work together, not only at the beginning, but also later on as you make your new life permanent. When it comes to attaining and maintaining your weight and fitness goals, what you eat and how you exercise are vital. But if you're relying only on your willpower and your ability to psych yourself up on the days when you're tired, hassled, rushed, or especially stressed out, you're likely to lose sight of the original vision. You need faith. Faith is like the electricity that powers the work you're doing on yourself. You can't see it, but you can feel its effects. In previous chapters we talked about how changing the way we think about our lives lays a solid foundation for the One-Day Way. With that foundation now in place, you're ready to begin construction on your new life. To do your best work, you need to see clearly what you're doing. You need the vision and power that faith supplies.

Have you ever driven on the highway late at night and seen crews working on repairs? They rig up huge, bright spotlights to enable them to see what they're doing. Obviously, they wouldn't get much done if they had to work in the dark. Faith is the electricity that provides the light you need to see what you're building, the juice to run your power tools, the energy that keeps you going.

You may not be a very religious person. But when I talk about the importance of faith, I'm not talking about religion. I'm talking about having faith that God loves you and wants you to have a healthy, fulfilling life. Also, you need to have faith in your ability to change. We all have the ability to make decisions that determine our actions. Better decisions lead to more-constructive actions. Give yourself some credit for being able to choose well, and be consistent in following through with the right actions. I'm also asking you to trust the simple, practical wisdom in the One-Day Way program. Changing your life in one day and then doing it again another day and another day after that sounds deceptively simple. It's tempting to think that it's so simple there's no way it can work. Don't weight-loss programs have to be burdensome and complicated to be effective? No. Think about the ones you've tried in the past and lost interest in. How much lasting good did they do?

So have some faith in the simplicity and lasting impact of this approach. You put faith in things every day. When you make a deposit at the bank, you trust the money will end up in your account. How about when you drop off your kids at school? It takes faith to believe they will be there when you go back to get them later in the day. Even something as simple as driving to the grocery store involves faith that your car will get you where you want to go.

IT'S TIME TO PLUG IN TO MORE POWER

When faith surges through us, we feel more alive. Faith is like electricity: when we have more of it, we have more power to "do" life with. Faith is the electrical current that charges our commitments. With increased faith we can take on new challenges, even the seemingly impossible ones.

God's power for your life is available, but you have to plug in to it. And remember, having faith is not the same as being religious. Putting your faith in God's love and trusting in His power is a decision you make, a commitment you base your life on. It has nothing to do with joining a religion.

I was getting my hair colored at the salon recently (sorry, I'm not a real blonde), and my hairdresser began to talk about some of his problems. Trying to be helpful, I responded with a question: "What's your faith like?" He quickly changed the subject, adding, "One of the very first things I learned in beauty school was never to discuss religion or politics." I didn't want to discuss either one. I just wanted to know if he believed things would get better. He thought I wanted to know whether he was Muslim or Catholic or Protestant. Just hearing the word *faith* is touchy for a lot of people.

Yet for others, faith is a way of life.

Without faith, Thomas Edison could never have devised the hundreds of major inventions he is credited with (the light bulb, phonograph, etc.). Without faith, the Wright brothers would never have tried to fly. Think about how much faith it must have taken to send a man to the moon. Or much more recently, consider the enormous amount of faith it must have taken to land a disabled commercial jetliner in the Hudson River. Faith seems a simple thing, yet our past mistakes often drag us down, hold us back, and keep us from tapping into its power.

As you begin to reconstruct your life, perhaps you don't have much faith in yourself because you let yourself down in the past. Let this go, and begin believing you are strong and have been designed with a purpose. Remember, the One-Day Way is all about starting fresh today. What happened yesterday, last week, or last year is past. It's finished. You're living today, and you have a chance every day to start over, to do things right, to make commitments and act on them. So let go of the past. It's the only way you'll be free to build your new life.

At times life will beat you up. You'll be so burdened, distracted, or stressed out that you can't seem to remember what you want or why. You'll lose sight of the new life you desire. Your vision will be clouded. Trust me, I still have those days. This is when the faith you have in something bigger than yourself is most important. When you find yourself lacking strength on your own, having faith in God's power can give you more energy than you could ever muster up yourself. This is because God is bigger than you and me, and He can see the entire picture of our lives.

Your Commitment Fueled by God's Help

I've never gone far when I've tried to rely on myself alone to accomplish something. But when I plug in to the power of my Creator, I find amazing, day-to-day strength to stay on course. On my journey to losing weight, I'd stop every day, sometimes every hour, and ask God to keep me strong and to help me press on, especially when I wanted a candy bar and had more faith in chocolate to satisfy me than in my commitment to live well, strong, and healthy.

Your measure of faith before this moment is unimportant. You may not feel as if you have a lot of faith, but it's important to remember that our feelings flow from our thinking. Whatever you decide to tell yourself can change your thinking, which in turn changes your feelings. You know this is true; part 2 of this book taught you how to change your thinking. You can do the same thing with faith. To plug in to that unseen power, start each day with a proclamation of faith. Here's one you can use when you wake up:

> Today I have faith that I have been designed with the ability to maintain self-control, to practice discipline, to speak only words that encourage, to be efficient with my time, and not to be distracted by anything or anyone who would interfere with my daily mission. I am meant to have a new life, and I will ask my Creator to help me do the things that will build that life today.

Saying these words every day is a faith-building exercise. When things get especially tough, you may need to recite this to yourself several times a day. Write it down, or type it into your phone and store it as a memo so it will be easily accessible. Faith will give you the energy to do the work that's necessary to break bad habits, make healthy choices, and say no to the people, influences, and temptations that would sabotage your success.

The commitments you've made, based on the power of faith, will drive your decisions when it comes to ordering lunch (salad or cheeseburger?) or hitting the treadmill (yes or no?). Once you begin to see results—when the number on your scale starts going down or you're less out of breath with exercise—your faith will grow. Faith gives you power to stick with it, and as you stick with it, you see more results. Then the results will encourage you and feed your faith. It's the most positive thing you can do as you rebuild your life.

You will need to have faith as you continue on the One-Day Way, because right now you can't see the end result. Practicing faith every day means living as if the choices you make will actually get you where you want to go. Circumstances will arise that may cause you to doubt what you're doing, and it will be a challenge to hold on to faith. But remember that faith is believing in something you can't see. You can't yet see the end result, but you will get there only by doing the necessary things for one day. And then again one day later.

From the start you will see bite-size results. You will take a thirty-minute walk when, in the past, you would have simply turned on the television. Or you will eat an apple instead of a slice of pie. Or you will avoid the office break room when you know someone has brought in pastries. It won't show the first day on your bathroom scale, but it will register in your mind and in your heart. You will know from the first day that you are a person who can make a commitment and keep it. And every small victory is cause for celebration.

Faith gets stronger with success. So don't forget to celebrate every success.

Chapter 11

Use Only High-Quality Materials

The One-Day Way to Eat

B y now you should feel charged up and eager to build new practices into your daily life. We will continue reconstructing your life by thinking differently about food. So far you have changed the way you think about the past and the future. You have let go of past failures and memories of doomed diets. You have freed yourself from the tyranny of a goal that's so far away it seems unattainable. You have dumped the discouragement and lack of confidence that have held you back. Now you are free from all that and have made the bedrock commitment to live better.

With a winning mind-set for changing your life, you're now ready to start reconstructing your body. While losing weight is only one part of changing your life, it's a crucial part. And it's the element that draws most people to the point of rebuilding their lives. Since every construction project needs material to build with, we're going to look at one of our most important building materials: food.

I'm not here to steal your sugary pleasures and to rob you of your rich, chocolate-filled happiness. But I am here to help you, for one day, think differently about food, be more knowledgeable about it, and begin to act differently around it. In this chapter you'll gain new information about the highest-quality building materials to reconstruct your life.

It's easy to think of food as the enemy or as something to avoid. But we all need to eat to make our bodies strong and healthy, so food is not our opponent. Instead, the enemy is our warped way of letting food control us.

On the other hand, food isn't *always* your friend. And it's never your best friend, the one who comforts you when you aren't given the promotion at work or when the guy you went out with didn't call you the next day or when your mother won't quit bugging you about your weight. That bowl of ice cream is not your best friend.

Do you remember the Dionne Warwick song about friendship? "For good times and bad times I'll be on your side forever more…"5 Listen up, friend. That's not what food is for! You must hear and own this truth to be set free so you can enjoy food in the future without being emotionally dependent on it.

Has food ever given you a solution in a time of crisis? Has food ever encouraged you to reach for the stars? Has food confronted you in a loving way when you were headed in the wrong direction? That's what real friends do, and I'm guessing food has probably not done any of those things for you. You should never turn to food for companionship, comfort, or a warm feeling inside.

It is, however, something you can and should enjoy. That's right: food should be thoroughly enjoyed on a regular basis. And it excites me to tell you the One-Day Way to eat will set you free from old guilt or worry about overindulging. It will also show you how to get maximum pleasure from food forever. I can make you a promise. At some point I will encourage you to eat the juiciest steak you can find. Then top it off with a slice of Key lime pie and whipped cream. Deal? But before we get there, we first need to look at how you value food.

It's Fuel, Not a Friend

Food is necessary for survival, which is why it's one of the most difficult addictions to control. The fear of not having enough food makes humans and animals do unthinkable things to protect their supply. People have reverted to animal behavior when there was a shortage of food. Hunger makes us feel desperate. We can't give up food entirely since we need it to sustain life. So we have to learn to use it as fuel for our bodies and enjoy it in moderation.

It's easy to get too attached to food. It tastes good, it promises to be our friend, and when we step away from it for a while, our stomach sends signals that cause us to obsess about needing a sandwich or a bagel. Look no further than the popular television series *Survivor* to see the effect that food deprivation has on people. This popular series puts a group of people in the wilderness and immerses them in crazy challenges to see who can survive in a difficult environment. The one who lasts the longest wins some serious cash. After having watched only a few episodes, I was intrigued by the lengths individuals will go to for nourishment. I saw one contestant eating centipedes and licking tree sap. This seems pretty desperate to me.

One recent episode got me thinking about the role of food in our lives.

We've all heard that we must eat to live instead of living to eat, right? I've said it countless times myself. I've even written these words in past books. But I've given more thought to this assumption and have revamped the familiar saying. What if we eat to live most of the time and then plan to live to eat occasionally? Let's make food the fuel for living but also have it be the center of attention at a celebration on rare occasions. That way we are choosing how to live rather than having food make all the calls for us. I find that when I mention this to people who love food, which seems to be most people, they don't immediately embrace the idea of eating to live. They start feeling robbed. They feel as though I'm taking away something that makes them happy. But with the right outlook, we can all eat to live and live to eat while feeling more in control of our choices.

It's a Gift, but Not Happiness

God gave us food as a gift. He could have made everything taste like a rice cake, but He didn't. He provided food with a variety of flavors and textures, colors and smells for us to enjoy. But there is a big difference between enjoying food and trying to maintain a friendship with it. You have to get clear on what food can give you and what it cannot. It can give you pleasure. It cannot give you emotional support. It can't be there for you when your dog dies.

One night on *Survivor* the contestants had to compete in a physical challenge for a prize. They had to stand on a log in the ocean to see who could keep their balance the longest. The winner got to enjoy a gourmet meal, which the producers had flown in. Naturally, the winner was elated. As I watched him eat each morsel, I wanted to cry (kind of). It was so beautiful to see him truly appreciate something delicious. He was savoring every bite as though he didn't want it to end. It was as if he had never tasted bread before.

You can enjoy food the same way, as if it's a rare delight. Even hot bread can taste like the nectar of the gods. But you can't enjoy food with that same intensity if every day you're indulging in rich, sugary, fatty foods. The One-Day Way food plan is designed to teach you to eat for survival most of the time, getting the maximum fuel from it and enjoying every bite, but not wasting calories with empty, nonnutritious food. As you take on challenges and keep a healthy perspective, you can look forward to the future opportunity to eat for pure reward and enjoyment. But on a day-to-day basis, food is fuel and not the meaning of life.

The problem with most people who struggle with food addiction or weight fluctuations is the stress of what to eat and when. For some reason many people feel they need constant variety to ward off boredom. They believe, wrongly, that food is meant for entertainment, a diversion along the lines of a crossword puzzle or a movie. In fact, diet companies and food-delivery programs pitch this idea. They want to sell you the dream that you can eat all your favorite foods and still lose weight. But boredom with food is sometimes necessary, because it robs food of its emotional power.

Most of us would not say that stopping at the gas station to fill the tank is a highlight of our day. Because your car needs fuel, you stop on the way home to gas up. It's not the most boring thing you do, but it's far from the most entertaining.

Mealtime is like that when you approach food primarily as fuel and not as prime-time entertainment. The other day I saw a kiosk in the mall selling products for "The Cookie Diet." Seriously. Apparently this diet says you can lose weight while eating cookies every day. I'm no genius, but does anyone think that people who love cookies so much they'd buy into a diet plan based on eating cookies are people who should be *encouraged* to eat cookies? The marketers of this diet are trying to get you to believe you don't need to give up anything to get the life you really want. And oh how I wish this were true.

Changing your life means giving up some things you're attached to. It might be cookies or soda pop or potato chips or veal. It's never easy. I know firsthand that letting go of something you love, even if it's for just a season, can feel like a death. However, when you learn to let go of foods that control you, there can be a rebirth. You can learn to have a completely different, healthy relationship with food when you're willing to let go of the way you loved food in the past. After you set new rules for your friendship with food, everything you have enjoyed can be brought back again, but in moderation.

When I set out to lose weight, my first goal was simply to exercise every day. Just to move for thirty minutes a day for the first month. At the beginning I didn't change my eating habits much, except I made a commitment to have breakfast every morning. And without exception, for the first month I made good on my commitment to exercise daily and to eat breakfast. There were days when I got my daily thirty minutes just before midnight, pacing around my cul-de-sac. But because I didn't try to tackle both exercise *and* cutting my food intake at the same time, I felt like I could manage it. And I did manage it. For the first time in years, I exercised every day. (If you're interested in hearing more about this, you can find it in my book *Never Say Diet.*)

Once the month was over, I decided to build on my success. In addition to continuing the thirty minutes of daily exercise, in the second month I decided to give up something related to food that tempted me. Day by day I said no to all sugary, processed foods. And I began to experience bite-size success each day.

From there, I moved on to predictable, three-hundred-calorie meals. I ate the same turkey sandwich with lettuce and tomato every day for almost six months. It's actually a very tasty sandwich, but I wouldn't call it exciting. But then, it didn't need to be exciting since I had decided that food was not my best friend, confidant, source of entertainment, or a shoulder to cry on. It was fuel.

So before we move on to the next chapter, in which we will learn the Ten Commandments of the One-Day Way to Eat for Weight Loss, let's accept that every meal doesn't need to be *va-va-va-voom* impressive. For me, drinking the same protein shake and having the same turkey sandwich every day for several months was a good thing. In fact, it was one of the best things I did when I began my self-designed journey. I never had to worry about what to fix for lunch, it was easy to do the grocery shopping, and I knew in advance how many calories I was consuming every day. Food was fuel, what I needed to survive. It wasn't a reward or a way to avoid being bored in the middle of the day. Once I realized that I wasn't going to die if I had the same thing for lunch every day and that eating boring meals didn't make me a boring girl, I had the freedom to begin to add some foods that were more pleasureful. But that came later, after I had rewritten the rules of my relationship with food. It was only then that I knew how to enjoy certain foods as a special delight and not as part of a daily attempt to entertain myself, fight off loneliness, or feed an unhealthy urge.

The meal plan for weight loss, which you'll find in chapter 13, is designed to help you lose weight in a healthy way. You'll eat 1,400 to 1,600 calories per day. With that calorie intake and following the suggested exercise plan in this book, you should be able to lose one or two pounds every week. If you're consuming an average of 1,500 calories a day and you aren't losing at least one pound per week, you may need to shave off 100 additional calories per day from your meal plan. Be sure to leave room for flexibility.

Also remember this: losing weight is not a scientific mystery. To take off weight, you must burn more calories than you take in. I know people try to make it more complicated than that, but it's not. The battle is in your thinking and your attitude. That's why the first part of this book was all about changing the way you think.

Now you will need to learn how to measure calories accurately. To do that, begin to read labels and to take time to measure amounts. Portions have become way too large in most restaurants and have distorted our view of proper serving sizes. So let's move on to the next chapter, where we'll begin to eat differently and become more knowledgeable about what we're eating.

. . . .

Chapter 12

The One-Day Way Food Rules

Ten Commandments for Weight Loss and for Life

To help you learn how to relate to food properly, here are the Ten Commandments of the One-Day Way to Eat for Weight Loss. Don't be afraid. The word *commandment* is not meant to be intimidating. You may think of a commandment as a restriction, but really it's a path to freedom. The Ten Commandments that God gave in the Bible were meant to be full of promise. If we keep them, we live purpose-filled lives, and we're protected from the harm that comes from unwise choices and actions. In the same way, the Ten Commandments of the One-Day Way to Eat for Weight Loss are full of promise. I have practiced them for years and experienced the rewards. Nearly nine years after I lost two hundred pounds, I'm still maintaining my target weight, working as a personal trainer, running marathons, and loving my new-found fitness. These rules for maximum nutrition are designed to help you get on course and stay on course with the role of food in your life.

One day at a time, you can lose the weight you need to lose—and then maintain a healthy weight for the rest of your life. You will also be set free from allowing food to control you ever again. Here are the rules.

THE TEN COMMANDMENTS OF THE ONE-DAY WAY TO EAT FOR WEIGHT LOSS

1. Consume 1,400 to 1,600 calories per day for weight loss, then 2,000 to 2,500 calories per day for life.
2. Never skip breakfast.
3. Maintain a balanced diet.
4. Eat six times per day.
5. Drink lots of water.
6. Be aware of portion size.
7. Learn how to snack smart.
8. Do a daily hunger check.
9. Fight fat with fiber.
10. Indulge one meal, one time per week. Fast one meal, one time per week.

Read the list again and think about it. Begin to think how the ten rules apply to your everyday life. Copy the list onto a card or sheet of paper, and post it where you'll see it every day. Consult the list when you're making decisions about what to eat or planning meals for the day.

The First Commandment

Consume 1,400 to 1,600 calories per day for weight loss, then 2,000 to 2,500 calories per day for life.

The first commandment will help free you from the stress of worrying about what you ate yesterday or what you will have tomorrow. Depending on where you are relative to your weight-loss goal, consume no more than 1,600 calories per day. To lose one pound of body fat, you must take away 3,500 calories. That means you'd have to burn 3,500 more calories than you ate in one day, which would be very difficult to do. However, if you take in 500 fewer calories per day than you need to fuel your daily activities, then over a week you would burn 3,500 more calories than you took in, and you would lose one pound. If you take in 1,000 fewer calories per day than you need to fuel your activities, then over a week you would burn 7,000 more calories than you took in and would lose two pounds.

Right now you might be thinking, *If I eat even less, I'll lose weight faster!* At first this is true. But if you're losing more than two pounds a week, you may be putting your body into starvation mode and ultimately slowing down your metabolism. Eventually your body will try to hang on to its reserves by slowing down as it also stores up. Just remember, in the first few weeks you can lose much more weight due to fluid loss, so you don't need to starve yourself.

The One-Day Way to Eat for Weight Loss is based on consuming 1,400 to 1,600 calories a day. This calorie amount is adequate to meet your nutrition needs while also giving you enough food that you won't feel deprived. An ongoing feeling of deprivation caused by dieting is a major cause for rebounding and regaining the weight. To avoid this, you'll combine this eating plan with the exercise plan in chapters 14 and 15.

You'll have to think about what you eat. Sorry, it's true. I recommend that for the first several weeks you carry a notepad to keep a record of your meals and the calorie totals for the day. You can make this really easy by finding several basic meals you enjoy and repeating them every day. The more basic you keep your meals and the more you repeat them, the less attention you'll have to pay to calculating calories. If you have the same few things for lunch each day, you have to calculate the calories less frequently.

At the end of the day, it's time to total up your calories. Celebrate whatever small successes you had. If you chose fruit instead of cookies, congratulations. If your total calorie intake was between 1,400 and 1,600, excellent. Then rip up the notes for that day. Tomorrow it won't matter. The One-Day Way to Eat is based on what you eat today. Tomorrow is another day, another chance to be healthy and fit. This breaks the pattern of feeling as if you've eaten too much and you should starve the next day. Or when you've eaten too little, you can no longer feel the following day should hold extra benefits, like an ice cream sundae.

Once you've reached your optimal weight, you'll shift from the plan for weight loss to the One-Day Way to Eat for Life. This second plan is based on 2,000 to 2,500 calories per day. The higher end of the range is meant more for men and extremely active people (those who exercise at least fifteen hours per week). I've found I can maintain my healthy weight range by eating approximately 2,200 calories daily and exercising. (I am extremely active.)

The Second Commandment
Never skip breakfast.

Don't even think about skipping breakfast! Why? First, breakfast revs your metabolism, the rate at which your body burns calories. You break the fast you've been on since your last meal the night before. Once you take in food, first thing, the engine (your metabolism) is restarted. I suggest you eat within two hours of waking up.

Second, breakfast delivers energy. When you begin your day with quality carbs and protein, you'll be sharp and ready for the day ahead. You don't have to eat a large quantity. Focus on quality of food, and be sure to get protein. (Hint: even though cheese has some protein, a cheese danish is *not* a good breakfast choice!)

Finally, breakfast helps prevent you from eating too much late at night. Most people who can't seem to lose weight say that's when they blow it. Naturally, as the mind and body slow down, they begin to process hunger signals more distinctly than they did during your busy day. If you've skipped meals and perhaps not taken in an adequate amount of calories, you are more likely to overeat late in the day or at night. And because you're getting tired, you're more likely to choose unhealthy food. The bottom line: breakfast is the key to feeling like a champion.

The Third Commandment
Maintain a balanced diet.

Our bodies need a variety of nutrients. A balanced diet has proper amounts of carbohydrates, protein, and fat. I know what you're thinking: *Aren't carbs bad? How much protein should I be eating, and what about eggs and cottage cheese? While we're at it, what's the deal with fat?* You can find more detailed information about nutrition on my Web site (www.chantelhobbs.com). For now, let's take a quick look at the most important things you need to know in creating a balanced diet.

First, carbohydrates are necessary. They're the building blocks of energy. But not all carbs are alike. Simple sugars (simple carbs), such as those found in cookies, candy, and fruit, enter the bloodstream quickly and give a rush of energy, followed by a "crash." Complex carbohydrates, found in foods such as potatoes, rice, oatmeal, and pasta, are digested more slowly and supply energy over a longer time. You should get about 40 percent of your daily calories from carbs, mostly complex carbs made with whole grains.

Protein should account for about 30 percent of your daily calorie total. Protein is vital to building and maintaining muscle. Remember, lean muscle is the backbone of a healthy metabolism. Because of the aging process, we all lose some muscle each year. This means strength training is important to maintaining not only your strength but also muscle mass. Be sure to choose protein that is lean, such as skinless chicken, skinless turkey, and fish, most of the time. You can also find nonmeat sources of protein in vegetables such as beans or in dairy products, including milk and yogurt.

A healthy, balanced diet also includes fat. Some fats, such as omega-3, are essential to brain development. You find omega-3 in foods such as salmon and walnuts. About 30 percent of your daily calories should come from fats. Steer clear of trans fats and hydrogenated oils, which are unhealthy and hard to digest. These are the ones found in many processed, prepackaged baked goods, and fast foods. Get your fat from fish, nuts, or plants (such as avocado). Avoid processed foods as much as possible.

The Fourth Commandment
Eat six times per day.

Eating six times throughout the day is important to maintaining your energy level and keeping your body well fueled. This does not mean you should consume a cheeseburger and fries every three hours. A meal is not a four-course dinner but simply giving your body some fuel. So don't get stressed thinking you need to cook or prepare complicated foods several times a day. Instead, keep healthy foods that nature has prepackaged near at hand. Good choices include fruits, vegetables, and nuts. If it helps, you can measure out small amounts into plastic bags or small containers. This will keep you from having to stop and think about what to eat next. I've found that most people who struggle with dinnertime and late-night snacking tend to deprive their bodies of an adequate amount of calories earlier in the day. So be sure you don't skip meals throughout the day. If for a few weeks you need to set an alarm on your cell phone as a reminder to eat an apple and some almonds at 11 a.m., go for it!

If you are on the One-Day Way to Eat for Weight Loss, you should be having about 1,500 calories per day. Here's an example of the calorie breakdown:

Breakfast: 350 calories

Midmorning snack: 200 calories

Lunch: 350 calories

Midafternoon snack: 150 calories

Dinner: 350 calories

Evening snack: 100 calories

Once you achieve your target weight, you'll shift to a maintenance meal plan. At that point you should consume about 2,000 calories per day. Here's an example of the calorie breakdown:

Breakfast: 400 calories

Midmorning snack: 250 calories

Lunch: 450 calories

Midafternoon snack: 250 calories

Dinner: 400 calories

Evening snack: 250 calories

Use these calorie breakdowns as a general guideline. Just remember, saving calories for rainy days doesn't work. Your body can only process and use what it needs a little at a time. Therefore, having only a few large meals a day can wreak havoc on your body's ability to keep you well energized. Grazing is the act of consuming little bits at a time. Begin to think of yourself as a grazer, and you'll feel great all day long.

The Fifth Commandment

Drink lots of water.

Did you know a human can survive a few weeks without food but without water will last only a few days? Our bodies are approximately 70 percent water.

Water is contained in our cells and bloodstream. The body's water supply is involved in nearly every bodily process. Water is required for the distribution of nutrients, electrolytes, hormones, and other chemical messengers, as well as in the removal of waste products. Water is involved in cellular energy production and the maintenance of body temperature. When you drink plenty of water, you cleanse your body of toxins, reduce sodium buildup, relieve constipation, and maintain proper muscle tone.

To determine how much water you should drink every day, take your body weight in pounds and divide it by two. This is the number of ounces of water you should drink in a day. So if you weigh 150 pounds, you should drink seventy-five ounces of water per day. If you weigh 200 pounds, drink a hundred ounces of water daily. Get a refillable water bottle and carry it with you, sipping from it all day.

Here's the formula: your weight (in pounds) divided by 2 = amount of water to drink (in ounces).

The Sixth Commandment

Be aware of portion size.

I can make you a promise: if you can control your portions, you can master weight control *forever.* Eating out usually presents the greatest challenge for someone trying to lose weight because restaurants want you to feel that you're getting your money's worth. The food on your plate doesn't cost them anywhere near what you pay for it. So to justify the menu price, they need to compensate by adding more to your plate. Keep telling yourself, *Just because there is still food on my plate, that doesn't mean I have to eat it!* Take half home, or simply leave it.

Don't allow your mother's old admonition that children are starving in China to guilt you into overeating. When you sit down to a meal, divide what is on your plate into three parts. First draw a line down the middle. One half of the plate should contain your salad and/or vegetables. Then divide the other half into two equal parts (each is one-quarter of the entire plate). One quarter should hold your protein (meat), and the other should supply the starch (pasta, rice, roll, potato). When you're dining out, if the portions provided don't match this ratio, ask for a second plate. Divide your food so the portion sizes are correct, and get the rest boxed to take home for another meal.

Also, begin to pay close attention to labels. Often the serving sizes aren't obvious. Just because you're buying a little bag of pretzels, don't assume that is one portion. When you read the fine print, you may discover that little bag has three servings in it! So the caloric content of one serving is actually tripled if you eat the entire small bag. Read labels to make informed choices about what you eat.

The Seventh Commandment
Learn how to snack smart.

I can't tell you how many times I've seen this dilemma: people tell me they're trying to lose weight by eating healthy and exercising but the number on the scale won't budge. What's usually happening is that they're consuming mindless calories. They're snacking and not counting the calories. They think, *What's one bite?* But if they take just one bite twenty times a day, they've added a full-size, calorie-laden snack to the day's food intake.

Here are tips to help you avoid this trap. For a while eat only when you're sitting down at a table (not sitting in front of the television). This will force you to slow down and think before you put something in your mouth. Also, when it comes to smart snacking, use the following list of Ten P Power Snacks. All the snacks on the list begin with the letter *P* to make them easier to remember. I created the list for my own benefit. I found that I'd been choosing a snack based on a craving for crunch, salt, or sweetness. But allowing a craving to make your decision is not a good way to lose weight.

This list has all three—crunchiness, saltiness, and sweetness. But when portioning, I'm careful to make the amount equal no more than 200 to 250 calories at one time. That lets me know I can have a lot more popcorn than peanuts for the same amount of calories. I always keep these snacks around, and most of them have some nutritional value. Of course, nothing is as good for snacking as raw fruits and veggies. However, the truth is that at times you want something that tastes more like a treat. Just try to do this in conjunction with eating a good supply of nutritious foods throughout the day to offset the occasional snack that may not be so good for you.

Some food manufacturers are selling 100-calorie packs. While this provides portion control, often the food is not very healthy. In almost every instance, eating packaged food is inconsistent with a healthy lifestyle. Reintroduce yourself to the produce section of the grocery store.

Chantel's Ten P Power Snacks

1. Peanuts
2. Pretzels
3. Pickles
4. Popsicles (sugar free)
5. Pudding (fat free)
6. Popcorn
7. Protein shakes
8. Protein bars
9. Pistachios
10. Potato chips (baked)

The Eighth Commandment

Do a daily hunger check.

The One-Day Way is all about making the best choices one day at a time. A major key to shedding pounds and not gaining them back is to know your body and your hunger levels.

At the age of two, my son Jake had me worried. There were days when it seemed like all he ate was the ketchup on a french fry. When I mentioned this to his pediatrician, he taught me the beauty of this commandment. He said that for the most part, children eat based on the signals their bodies give them. He told me not to worry and not to push Jake to eat but just to offer him healthy food. When a growth spurt comes, the doctor assured me, he will eat everything in sight. Boy, was the doctor right. Since that time, I've always tried to make my kids do hunger checks. When they ask for a snack or something to eat, I want to know if they're truly hungry or simply bored and looking for something to do. Many of us never stop to ask ourselves that question.

I don't want to confuse you since I've already told you to eat several small meals throughout the day. But as you do that, remember that as you begin to run your body more like a machine, you'll know what it needs and when. The daily hunger check will remind you that you don't always need to eat something just because it's been a few hours since your last meal. To lose weight, you'll need to experience some form of deprivation regularly. Otherwise your body won't be able to use excess fat. I know that may be difficult to hear, but it's true.

Here's how to do a hunger check. When you start to feel hungry, rate it on a scale of one to five. Then follow my advice for each level of hunger.

Level 1: "I think I might be getting a little hungry, but I just ate an hour ago." You're not hungry. Stop thinking about food, and go fold some laundry.

Level 2: "I need something to eat soon. It's been a few hours since I ate last.

I'm feeling kind of tired." Drink a glass of water, eat an apple, and have a handful of almonds.

Level 3: "I'm starving. I would do *anything* for food!" You're entering a danger zone. Always have something on hand, such as a protein bar, for these times. Protein satisfies longer than fruit. Also, having some hummus and pretzels can help at a time like this.

Level 4: "I'm going to start chewing on my arm or eat someone else's arm." You've gone too long without food. You need to have at least 300 calories of protein and carbs immediately! Do it now!

Level 5: "Hand over the chips, some cookies, and a bowl of ice cream!" All I can say is, watch out! This means you ignored every signal your body sent, and now you're about to jump ship. Stop and think about how this happened so you can avoid it in the future. Next, stop and sit down to a solid meal. If you can't make this happen immediately, eat a granola bar, a handful of peanuts, and an orange. Then, as soon as possible, have a big salad and a piece of chicken.

The Ninth Commandment
Fight fat with fiber.

If there were one big secret to weight loss, fiber would be it! Most people realize that fiber, or roughage, is necessary for good digestion. I'm just not convinced that people fully understand the tremendous benefits of fiber. First of all, fiber curbs your appetite because it makes you feel full. Think about eating a doughnut for breakfast or having a bowl of oatmeal. Naturally, the oatmeal will stick with you because it's fiber rich. Also, a high-fiber diet cleanses the intestines and removes wastes, even fat, more quickly. This process will take some ingested fat along with it.

The greatest benefit received from a high-fiber diet is the steady level of insulin it produces. Because fiber evens out your insulin levels, you're able to burn fat more efficiently. When you experience a sugar rush, or big fluctuations in insulin from consuming too many simple sugars, your body tends to store fat more readily. Here's the bottom line: consume twenty-five to thirty grams of fiber a day.

The Tenth Commandment

Indulge one meal, one time per week. Fast one meal, one time per week.

This last commandment is the most exciting and most rewarding. Remember the gourmet meal I told you about earlier that was given to the winner of a competition on *Survivor*? This is going to be you, once a week. Make it a point one time every week to eat for pure enjoyment. I'm not talking about hitting every Chinese buffet in town, followed by a Dairy Queen marathon. I'm saying, plan and enjoy a meal with someone, or several people, you really care about. And do it once a week. Don't be in a hurry to finish the meal. Whether it's at a restaurant or you prepare it yourself, indulge with the mind-set of living to eat just for the moment. Savor this meal; truly enjoy it.

Doing this once a week reminds us that food should not be a source of punishment and guilt but that it can be fun and full of pleasure.

There is one other food-related habit to practice weekly. For one meal go on a fast. By letting go of a meal, whichever one you choose, you will be controlling your hunger and also practicing self-discipline. Both of the weekly practices—indulging and fasting—are important to losing weight and then maintaining your target weight. You know in advance that you can indulge in and really enjoy great food, and then you can switch back to being in control of your desires.

By practicing both of these, you'll have the One-Day Way to Eat for Weight Loss system down. You will get maximum benefit from food, enjoy it more, and look better than you have in years.

. . . .

Chapter 13

How to Eat Cleaner, Beginning Today

Meal Plans That Make a Difference

It's much easier to stick to a plan of consuming 1,400 to 1,600 calories per day, eating six meals per day, if you have a simple meal plan to follow. Here are two one-week meal-plan examples to help you get started. You'll notice these are basic meals that require little preparation. You'll also have chances to prepare extravagant recipes, especially if cooking is something you love to do.

However, if you're anything like me, most days your schedule is crowded, and you need simple dishes that will work for your entire family. You may have to change some of your previous eating habits. For example, I had to stop making casseroles, which often are loaded with calories and salt. I had to learn to make clean, simple, healthy meals, like the ones in these plans.

These meal plans give you food that tastes good, is filling, delivers maximum fuel, and has main ingredients that are easy to keep on hand. It simplifies shopping and meal preparation, freeing up time for exercise and other things you enjoy.

THE ONE-DAY WAY TO EAT FOR WEIGHT LOSS

Here is a one-week meal plan for weight loss. It supplies approximately 1,500 calories per day.

Day 1

Breakfast: 1 cup Kashi GOLEAN cereal, 1 cup skim milk; ½ banana; 1 tablespoon peanut butter

Midmorning snack: 1 cup low-fat cottage cheese; 1 cup blueberries

Lunch: Turkey sandwich: 2 slices whole-wheat bread, 2 deli-style slices turkey, 1 slice low-fat cheese, tomato, lettuce, onion, dab of fat-free mayo, dab of mustard; 1 medium apple

Midafternoon snack: 1 cup low-fat vanilla yogurt, 1 tablespoon granola; 1 hard-boiled egg

Dinner: 4 ounces grilled salmon; ½ baked sweet potato, dash of cinnamon, 1 tablespoon brown sugar; 1 cup steamed broccoli

Evening snack: 10 strawberries, 2 tablespoons chocolate Reddi-wip

Day 2

Breakfast: 1 packet instant oatmeal, 1 tablespoon chopped walnuts, 1 tablespoon raisins; 2 slices turkey bacon

Midmorning snack: Scrambled eggs (4 whites plus 1 whole egg); ½ grapefruit

Lunch: 4 ounces grilled skinless chicken breast; ½ cup brown rice; 1 cup green beans

Midafternoon snack: 2 cups light butter popcorn; 2 deli-style slices turkey

Dinner: 4 ounces lean sirloin burger (grilled or broiled), ½ whole-wheat bun, 1 tablespoon ketchup or mustard; 1 ear of boiled or grilled corn; ½ cup steamed peas

Evening snack: 10 pretzels, 2 tablespoons hummus

Day 3

Breakfast: Strawberry-banana protein shake: 1 small banana, 5 small strawberries, 1 scoop vanilla protein powder, 8 ounces water, ½ cup ice, 1 tablespoon honey. Blend all ingredients.

Midmorning snack: 1 fat-free string cheese stick; 1 nectarine; 3 deli-style slices turkey

Lunch: Tuna wrap: 3 ounces white tuna packed in water, 1 table-spoon each chopped celery and carrots, 1 tablespoon fat-free mayo, 1 tablespoon low-fat plain yogurt. Mix all ingredients, then put the mixture into a whole-wheat wrap. Add 10 grapes on the side.

Midafternoon snack: ½ whole-wheat English muffin, 1 tablespoon peanut butter, 1 tablespoon all-fruit jam

Dinner: ½ roasted chicken, white meat only; ½ cup brown rice; ½ cup black beans; tossed salad, 2 tablespoons fat-free or light dressing; veggies

Evening snack: 2 sugar-free Popsicles

Day 4

Breakfast: ½ whole-wheat bagel, 2 tablespoons fat-free cream cheese; 2 deli-style slices lean honey ham

Midmorning snack: 1 orange; ¼ cup raw unsalted almonds

Lunch: Tomato-and-cheese sandwich: 2 slices whole-wheat bread, 2 slices reduced-fat cheddar cheese, 4 thick slices beefsteak tomato, mustard; 1 small pear

Midafternoon snack: Granola bar; 2 deli-style slices lean roast beef

Dinner: Chicken Caesar salad: romaine lettuce, 4 ounces grilled skinless chicken breast, 2 tablespoons light Caesar dressing, 2 tablespoons parmesan cheese

Evening snack: 2 cups light kettle corn popcorn

Day 5

Breakfast: Peach protein shake: 1 cup low-fat peach yogurt, 1 scoop vanilla protein powder, ½ peach (cut up), 6 ounces water, ½ cup ice. Blend all ingredients.

Midmorning snack: Celery sticks, carrot sticks, 2 tablespoons light ranch dressing; 1 cup cantaloupe

Lunch: Barbecued open-faced chicken sandwich: 4 ounces grilled skinless chicken, 1 tablespoon barbecue sauce, 1 slice whole-wheat bread, lettuce, tomato, onion; 1 medium apple

Midafternoon snack: 10 walnuts; 10 grapes

Dinner: Southwestern salad: ½ cup black beans, ½ cup low-salt canned corn, ½ cup brown rice, 1 tablespoon salsa, 1 teaspoon chopped cilantro

Evening snack: ½ cup frozen vanilla yogurt, 1 tablespoon granola

Day 6

Breakfast: ¾ cup raisin bran cereal, 1 cup skim milk; 2 slices turkey bacon

Midmorning snack: 8 ounces low-fat plain yogurt, 1 tablespoon honey, 1 tablespoon almonds, 1 tablespoon cranberry raisins

Lunch: Peanut butter and jelly wrap: 1 whole-wheat tortilla, 1 tablespoon peanut butter, 1 tablespoon all-fruit jam; ½ banana

Midafternoon snack: 1 cup skim milk with 2 teaspoons chocolate syrup; 1 low-fat graham cracker

Dinner: Shrimp-and-veggie pasta: 1 cup whole-wheat pasta, ½ package steamed mixed vegetables (broccoli and carrots), 10 medium shrimp sautéed in 1 tablespoon olive oil and garlic. Mix all ingredients with salt and pepper. Add 1 tablespoon parmesan cheese on top.

Evening snack: 10 frozen grapes, 2 tablespoons low-fat Reddi-wip

Day 7

Breakfast: Salsa scramble: 1 egg plus 2 egg whites scrambled in a pan coated with nonstick spray, 2 tablespoons salsa, 1 tablespoon fat-free shredded cheese; 1 whole-wheat English muffin, 1 tablespoon all-fruit jam

Midmorning snack: 20 almonds, 10 strawberries

Lunch: Turkey raspberry roll-up: 1 whole-wheat tortilla, 1 tablespoon raspberry jam, 1 slice reduced-fat cheese, 3 ounces roasted turkey breast

Midafternoon snack: 2 tablespoons hummus, 20 pretzels

Dinner: 4 thin slices lean pork tenderloin; 1 cup squash, 1 cup zucchini steamed and tossed in 1 tablespoon olive oil; 1 small potato with salt and pepper to taste

Evening snack: 10 strawberries, 2 tablespoons low-fat Reddi-wip

THE ONE-DAY WAY TO EAT FOR LIFE

Here's a one-week meal plan to follow after you've achieved your target weight. This plan supplies approximately 2,000 calories per day. At that calorie level, as long as you're getting regular exercise, you should be able to maintain your weight for a lifetime.

Day 1

Breakfast: 2 frozen whole-grain waffles, ½ cup strawberries, 1 table-spoon chopped walnuts, 1 tablespoon real maple syrup

Midmorning snack: 1 apple; ½ cup sunflower seeds

Lunch: Chef salad: salad/veggies; 4 ounces deli turkey (cut up), 1 slice reduced-fat cheese (cut up), 1 ounce low-sodium ham (cut up), 1 hard-boiled egg (cut up), 2 tablespoons light ranch dressing

Midafternoon snack: 15 reduced-fat tortilla chips, ½ cup salsa

Dinner: 1 cup whole-wheat pasta, 1 cup meat sauce, 1 tablespoon parmesan cheese; tossed salad, 1 tablespoon light Italian dressing; 1 cup sautéed spinach

Evening snack: 1 fat-free pudding cup, 1 cup frozen blueberries, 2 tablespoons light whipped cream

Day 2

Breakfast: 2 hard-boiled eggs; ½ cup steamed spinach; 1 whole-wheat English muffin toasted; 1 cup cantaloupe

Midmorning snack: Granola bar; ½ banana; 1 cup low-fat cottage cheese

Lunch: Ham-and-cheese roll-up: 4 ounces low-fat ham, 1 slice low-fat cheese, 1 whole-wheat tortilla; 1 tangerine

Midafternoon snack: 1 slice whole-wheat bread, 2 tablespoons peanut butter, 1 tablespoon honey; ½ banana sliced

Dinner: 4 ounces grilled skinless chicken breast; ¾ cup couscous; 1 cup broccoli; 1 cup pineapple

Evening snack: 2 cups light kettle corn popcorn; 1 chocolate chip cookie

Day 3

Breakfast: 2 slices whole-wheat toast, 1 tablespoon almond butter; 1 medium pear

Midmorning snack: Chocolate protein shake: 1 scoop chocolate protein powder, 1 teaspoon chocolate syrup, 1 cup skim milk, ½ cup ice. Mix in blender.

Lunch: Large tuna salad: Mixed lettuce, onion, tomatoes, peppers, ½ cup garbanzo beans, 3 ounces tuna packed in water, 2 tablespoons reduced-fat salad dressing; 2 crisp bread crackers; 1 apple

Midafternoon snack: ½ cup unsalted soy nuts

Dinner: 1 slice cheese pizza with veggies; 1 large mixed salad, 1 tablespoon light Italian dressing; 1 cup mixed fruit

Evening snack: 1 cup skim milk; 1 *biscotto*

Day 4

Breakfast: 1 cup raisin bran cereal, 1 cup skim milk; 1 banana; 1 hard-boiled egg

Midmorning snack: ½ English muffin, 1 tablespoon peanut butter

Lunch: 2 cups low-sodium minestrone soup; 6 crackers; 3 slices grilled skinless chicken breast

Midafternoon snack: 1 cup vanilla soy milk; 1 peach

Dinner: 4 ounces mahimahi pan-seared in olive oil; 1 medium sweet potato, 1 teaspoon butter; 1 cup broccoli; 1 cup coleslaw made with shredded cabbage and 2 teaspoons of fat-free mayo, pepper

Evening snack: 3 cups low-fat popcorn

Day 5

Breakfast: 1 whole-grain bagel, 2 teaspoons low-fat cream cheese; 2 hard-boiled eggs

Midmorning snack: 1 cup low-fat vanilla yogurt, 2 tablespoons granola

Lunch: Turkey-and-veggie pita: 4 ounces turkey breast, 1 whole-wheat pita, 1 tablespoon fat-free mayo, lots of veggies; 1 oatmeal-raisin cookie

Midafternoon snack: 1 cup cantaloupe; ½ cup whole raw walnuts

Dinner: 4 ounces lean grilled sirloin; 1 small baked potato, 2 tablespoons fat-free sour cream; 1 cup steamed spinach sautéed in 1 tablespoon olive oil

Evening snack: ½ cup frozen strawberry yogurt

Day 6

Breakfast: Chocolate, peanut butter, banana smoothie: 1 scoop chocolate protein powder, 1 tablespoon peanut butter, ½ banana, ½ cup skim milk, 6 ounces water, ½ cup ice. Blend all ingredients.

Midmorning snack: ½ cup raw almonds; 1 orange

Lunch: 2 cups low-sodium chicken noodle soup; 6 crackers; 1 medium apple

Midafternoon snack: 1 large rice cake; 1 slice low-fat cheddar cheese; 3 deli-style slices low-fat chicken

Dinner: 4 ounces lean pork tenderloin; ½ cup wild rice; ½ cup snow peas; ½ cup carrots; small whole-wheat roll

Evening snack: 15 reduced-fat tortilla chips, ½ cup salsa

Day 7

Breakfast: 1 cup Kashi Good Friends cereal, 1 cup skim milk, 5 strawberries (cut up); 2 slices turkey bacon

Midmorning snack: ¼ cup sunflower seeds; 1 medium banana

Lunch: Roast beef and swiss wrap: 4 ounces lean roast beef, 1 slice reduced-fat swiss cheese. Place beef and cheese on whole-wheat wrap; warm in microwave for 20 seconds. Add 1 tablespoon spicy mustard, lettuce, tomato. Add 1 pear on the side.

Midafternoon snack: ½ cup frozen chocolate yogurt

Dinner: ¼ roasted white-meat, skinless chicken breast; 1 cup couscous; 1 cup steamed squash and zucchini drizzled in olive oil and seasoned with garlic salt

Evening snack: 3 tablespoons hummus, 20 pretzels; 1 cup vanilla soy milk

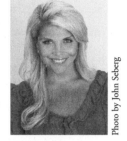

Photo by John Seberg

Chantel, how do you get your kids to eat vegetables?

I trick them. Sometimes I add veggies (diced or puréed) to pasta sauce and scrambled eggs. These days my kids get excited about "create a salad night," when they get to design their own salad and pick all the toppings. The goal is to get them to add in one new veggie they wouldn't usually choose!

Are all fast-food restaurants bad?

No! In fact, more fast-food establishments are offering healthy alternatives. The key is to look up the nutrition facts and be aware of exactly what's in the food you're ordering. Also, find ways to order less or eat less of what you order so you can cut down on portions. For example, when getting a grilled chicken sandwich, take off half the bun. This saves about 150 calories!

Is there a best time to do my weekly one-meal fast?

Yes. Fast for the meal that is the most challenging to give up. For me, breakfast wouldn't be hard to give up since it's not the meal I most look forward to. So I don't generally chose this meal to be a time of fasting. (Dinner is my favorite meal of the day.) Remember, the purpose of the fast is to remind you that food doesn't control you; you control it. So for a fast to have maximum impact, it needs to be challenging and uncomfortable.

Can I be a vegetarian and follow the One-Day Way of eating?

Absolutely. Let me say, adhering to a vegetarian lifestyle takes commitment. The most important thing is to make sure you get enough protein each day. To do this, drink protein shakes and eat eggs, nuts, peanut butter, and cheese often. Just be careful not to let cheese pizza become your main staple!

Which protein bars and protein shakes are best?

This is a great question. There are so many protein bars and shakes to choose from, it can be confusing. Be sure to pick a bar that contains around 200 calories and less than thirty grams of carbs. As for protein powder, select one that contains less than 150 calories per scoop and has at least twenty grams of protein.

I love your meal plan because it lets me indulge once a week. But I'm nervous that after I do that, I'll begin to crave bad foods again. Is this a danger?

Awesome question. The one meal each week when you indulge shouldn't scare you. However, if you feel this way, you could do your one-meal fast at the meal that follows. Also, if you choose to eat a large amount of "bad" food for the indulgent meal, you may find that you will feel terrible afterward. If this happens, use it as a reminder that you are now regularly eating healthy and feeling great as a result. This will help ensure you don't go back to giving in to your old cravings. Remember, the one meal per week when you indulge is designed to be a time for you to eat foods you enjoy but don't have on a regular basis.

Kelly's One-Day Way Story

All my life I've been a person who takes care of others. While that can be a generous thing to do, I can see that one reason I took on the caretaker role was to avoid facing my own problems.

When I was about eleven years old, my parents divorced. Whether I was happy, sad, scared, or lonely, I would eat. It wasn't easy to find ways to overeat. My mom didn't keep junk food in the house, so I would eat peanut butter straight out of the jar with a spoon. Eating was a way to soothe myself. But I was not extremely fat, so people didn't realize I was emotionally dependent on food.

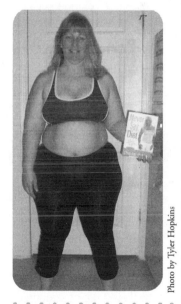

Photo by Tyler Hopkins

Over the years I've struggled with my weight, my finances, and more. I finally realized that the root issue of both my financial and physical problems was emotional. I'd occasionally try to do something about my weight. In June 2004, despite the fact that I was still 80 pounds overweight, I completed the one-hundred-mile Team in Training bike ride in Lake Tahoe in support of the Lymphoma/Leukemia Society. Six months later I ran the Disney Marathon, which is the regulation 26.2 miles. (I was still 80 pounds overweight.) I didn't do all the training I should have, and afterward I didn't stick with running. My eating problems and financial problems were still not resolved. But the best thing about training for the marathon was that I met Chantel, because she was a part of the Leukemia Society team with me.

We became friends, and she became my mentor. She took me and my son under her wing and made us feel a part of her family. She took me to church and helped me change my life. I was amazed at how she had lost 200 pounds while raising four kids. But even more than being impressed by her accomplishments, I was impressed by who she was.

At the point I met her, I was up to 272 pounds again. I knew it was time to change my life, but I still wanted to eat what was in front of me more than I wanted to lose weight. Eventually Chantel got tired of hearing me complain about my weight. She lovingly but very firmly said she'd had enough and that I could call to talk about anything *except* my weight problem. She said she didn't want to hear about it until I was ready to do something about it.

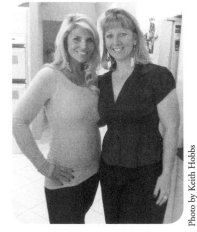

Photo by Keith Hobbs

I was having health issues by that time, including high cholesterol and achy joints. I was depressed and lonely and sick and tired of being sick and tired! I got so desperate to do something that I filled out paperwork to be on *The Biggest Loser*. My mom and family were supportive, and so was Chantel, but she said to me, "You know, Kelly, you can do this on your own!" I knew she was right.

In January 2008 I began the journey back to wellness. Chantel had given me a copy of her book *Never Say Diet,* and I started on her plan. I started eating healthy and began an exercise plan that included walking and strength training. I dropped from a size 24 to a size 10 to 12.

It feels good not only to lose weight but to be this fit. In April 2009, right after my fortieth birthday, I ran the Nashville half marathon. My next goal is to run the Disney Goofy in 2010, which is a half marathon on Saturday, followed by a full marathon on Sunday.

One of the greatest things about my new lifestyle is that I can do things with my son. We ride bikes together, and I even helped coach his football team. We recently ran our first 5K together, which was awesome. He's only eleven. He told me that he's happy that when he hugs me, his arms now reach all the way around.

If it were not for my faith in God, my family, my son Tyler, my friends, and especially Chantel, I would not be in this happy place in my life. I am grateful to all of them.

I now try to live one day at a time, with purpose. I focus on being the best I can be. I am trusting that God, who loves me, will help me be the best I can be every moment.

· ·

Chapter 14

Getting the Right Tools

Ten Commandments to Be Fit for Life

I enjoy shopping unless it involves a home-improvement store. But not too long ago, my husband coerced me into going to Home Depot for him. He needed a certain tool to complete a project I had asked him to do—adding an extra shelf to my closet. Since I really wanted that space to store the shoes I never wear, I headed off to Home Depot.

As I was leaving the house, I reminded Keith to keep a phone close by. I told him that his sending me to "that place" would be like my sending him to the Estée Lauder counter to pick up lip gloss. In other words, I was certain I'd be confused and lost.

As I had feared, when I got to the hammer aisle, I immediately saw that all the hammers looked exactly the same. I knew this couldn't be true. Why would there be so many different kinds if they were actually the same? Unless it's a hammer conspiracy designed to keep us girlie girls out of the way and off the testosterone-filled aisles?

I called Keith on my cell phone, and he walked me through the process of picking up the tools he needed. Of course I also had to put the hardware guy on the phone with him. Three times to be exact.

When I got home, I asked my husband why there are so many tools that seem like they would all get the same job done. And his response: it's mostly a matter of what you know works and what you like best.

The same is true for the tools you will use to reconstruct your life. To rebuild your body, you must use the tool of fitness. But there are many ways to get fit. In this chapter I'll show you a number of different fitness tools, and you can use the ones you like best.

My first time on an elliptical machine, I was completely out of breath in five minutes. Today I'm a marathon runner. I've tried many different types of physical training, and after nine years I know what works. Also, I have some preferences about the mental tools that put us in the right mind-set to get fit. Soon I'll be sharing them with you.

You can't skip the fitness part if you want to reconstruct your life. You have to balance your intake of food with activity that burns the fuel. So exercise is crucial. As with any exercise plan, you should talk to your doctor before you get started.

A woman came up to me after one of my speaking engagements a few years ago and asked, "Could you please tell me one exercise that will work the best to help me get into shape?" Without hesitating, I said, "There is just one, my friend." She looked around as if I were about to let her in on a very special secret. I leaned in and whispered, "Girl, it's the one you do every day."

The look on her face was priceless! Exercise is all about the moment. Sure, compounded over time, training will transform and tone your body. But the most important, results-giving principle to repeat to yourself is this: *Show up, show up. No matter what, keep on showing up.*

In *Never Say Diet* I wrote about my journey to fitness. It all began in a gym on a special recumbent bike. My goal each day was to show up and stay on that thing for thirty minutes. I did it six days a week for a solid month. And trust me, I got in and out of there in thirty-one minutes flat! But what I found out was that my daily goal was all that really mattered. Each time I showed up, no matter what, I was moving a little further ahead.

Now, nearly nine years later, not much has changed. Well, a few things have. Sure, now I'm a personal trainer, Spinning instructor, and marathon runner. All of which required long-term planning and learning some specific skills. But to achieve each of them, I still concerned myself with only one thing. Every day I asked myself, *What do I need to do* today *to get me closer to the next thing?* And while the "next thing" has changed many times, those things still are part of the lifestyle I have established. A life built on a daily, irrevocable commitment to optimal health.

In chapter 12 I gave you the Ten Commandments of the One-Day Way to Eat for Weight Loss. Changing your eating habits is essential, but it can't do the job alone. You need a second set of commandments, which are tools to reconstruct your body and your life. If you practice these commandments, you will look great and feel incredible for years to come.

THE TEN COMMANDMENTS OF THE ONE-DAY WAY TO GET FIT FOR LIFE

1. A great attitude isn't enough.
2. Believe that you were made to move.
3. Break a sweat every day.
4. Five days of cardio every week is nonnegotiable.

5. Intensity is important.

6. Something is better than nothing.

7. Results are a measure of personal progress.

8. Strength training three times a week is essential.

9. Recovery is required.

10. Figure out how to love exercise.

The First Commandment

A great attitude isn't enough.

Wouldn't it be nice if attitude really was everything? If all you had to do was believe superhard that all your goals would become reality and then, *poof,* they happened? Unfortunately the saying "Attitude is everything" is a pipe dream! Sure, I know that without a winning attitude you won't accomplish much. But taking regular *action* is just as important. If your new attitude doesn't produce consistent action, it's useless.

As you get your head in the right mind-set to tackle fitness one day at a time, remember attitude *and* action are all you need. First, wake up and believe you physically can do more than you were able to do the day before. Then add showing up to this, and *bam!* You begin to feel amazing at the end of every day. Begin with attitude and action; the results will astound you.

The Second Commandment

Believe that you were made to move.

Take a good look in the mirror, and check out the design of your arms and legs. Do you recognize they work best together? Try taking a walk and using only your legs—keeping your arms dangling at your sides. Do this for a minute or so. Next, lift your arms and engage them. Walk while pumping your arms. Not only will you move faster, but it's also easier. When you discover the design of your amazing body and realize that moving is a main feature, it will make you want to do it more often.

The Third Commandment
Break a sweat every day.

We will soon be talking about the One-Day Way to do cardio and strength training, but first, think *sweat*! Sweat is a bodily function that eliminates toxins. Regular sweating releases junk your body is holding, and it also makes you feel recharged and fresh. Well, maybe after a shower! Even if it's your day off from cardiovascular exercise, the One-Day Way is still based on breaking a sweat seven days every week. So if it's an "off day," find something to do for at least ten minutes that involves sweating. Here are a few suggestions: rake leaves, clean the swimming pool, shut off the air conditioning before you sweep and mop the floors, run up and down some stairs. You get the idea!

The Fourth Commandment
Five days of cardio every week is nonnegotiable.

You need to do cardiovascular exercise for two major reasons. One, to condition your heart muscle. By regularly doing cardio and getting your heart rate up for a period of time, you're forcing the heart muscle to become stronger, and a strong heart is more efficient in delivering oxygen-rich blood to your system. The second reason for cardio exercise is to burn calories more efficiently. Last week's three-mile run on the treadmill doesn't burn a single calorie for you today. You need to elevate your heart rate five days every week.

A hundred years ago a much larger percentage of the population was engaged in manual labor on farms and in other work settings. More people were active in the course of an ordinary workday. Let's face it, there isn't as much farming happening these days! Most people have jobs and daily responsibilities that don't involve a lot of motion. The amount of calories you burn just "doing life" is dramatically less than it was for your great-grandparents. Trust me, they didn't need an elliptical machine to lose weight. Most likely they just ran to the well a few more times to fill the water bucket. It's ironic that we have all these gadgets designed to save time and make our lives easier, and because of them, we now have to schedule sweating! It's a little silly but true.

So for a minimum of five days a week, do thirty minutes of some form of cardiovascular exercise. Cardio is any movement that keeps your heart pumping the entire time you're doing the activity. You'll find a list of cardio suggestions at the end of this chapter.

The Fifth Commandment
Intensity is important.

Pay very close attention to what I'm about to share with you. Intensity is what separates people who just work out from people who actually *get results* from their workouts! I can't count the number of people who tell me about their frustration with not getting results from exercise. Some have said, "I've walked five miles a day for the past several years, and I still see no changes." I tell them, "Show me your intensity." And nearly always the heart rate they're maintaining while doing their walk isn't much higher than it would be if they were strolling through the mall.

The intensity of your workouts is almost as important as your food choices. Here's why. Your body will adjust to an exercise that seems challenging initially and will learn how to do it with much less exertion. Therefore, a daily five-mile jaunt can begin to feel like a cakewalk unless you regularly increase your speed, choose a new route that involves steeper hills, alternate jogging with walking, carry light weights as you walk, or add other variations that ramp up the intensity.

By adding variations you can make a simple, five-mile walk an interval session. The definition of intervals is when you increase your work effort and follow it with a recovery (catch your breath) period. You should add interval training to your cardio sessions at least two times each week. The next page of this chapter has a sample interval session. Have fun making up some of your own.

The Basics of Interval Training

Use this interval session to get you jump-started. Interval training is the best way to increase intensity in your cardio workouts, and it burns a lot more calories. Intervals work well with any exercise you're able to do, and they don't add more time to the exercise session. Wearing a stopwatch helps.

On the sample interval session below, notice that the elapsed time (in minutes) for each work effort and recovery has a number next to it. The number coincides with a level of intensity, which helps make the intervals more measurable. Also, look at the perceived exertion scale before you start so you can gauge your workout accordingly.

Levels of Perceived Exertion

Levels 1–3:	"Hey, working out isn't so bad. I'm just warming up."
Level 4:	"This is not so easy. Is that a bead of sweat starting to run down my forehead?"
Level 5:	"Why are my legs starting to burn?"
Level 6:	"Yes! I'm sweating and feeling a little winded. Looks like I'll have to wash my hair when this is over!"
Level 7:	"I need to slow down for a second and catch my breath."
Level 8:	"Who says exercise is fun? I'm dying here!"

Level 9:   "I think I might throw up!"

Level 10:   "Someone put a fork in me. I'm officially cooked, done!"

A 30-Minute Interval Session

Minutes 1–5:   Work from a level 1 up to 3.

Minute 6:   Level 4.

Minute 7:   30 seconds at level 5; 30 seconds at level 6.

Minute 8:   30 seconds at level 7; 30 seconds at level 8.

Minute 9:   15 seconds at level 9; 45 seconds at level 4.

Minute 10:   Level 6.

Minutes 11–13:   Level 7.

Minute 14:   Level 8.

Minute 15:   30 seconds at level 5; 30 seconds at level 6.

Minute 16:   15 seconds at level 9; 45 seconds at level 4.

Minutes 17–19:   Level 7.

Minute 20:   Level 8.

Minute 21:   30 seconds at level 9; 30 seconds at level 4.

Minutes 22–23:   Recover down from level 4 to level 2.

Minute 24:   Level 4.

Minute 25:   Level 6.

Minute 26:   Level 7.

Minutes 27–28:   Level 8.

Minute 29:   45 seconds at level 6; 15 seconds at level 9.

Minute 30:   45 seconds at level 4; 15 seconds at level 9.

Cool down for 5 minutes.

The Sixth Commandment

Something is better than nothing.

Just after preaching to you about the importance of intensity, I need to remind you of a principle that will make all the difference in maintaining fitness. Hour-long intense workouts aren't always going to be possible, but something is still better than nothing. I maintain a hectic travel schedule and juggle being a wife and mother. There are times when the sky appears to be falling, and there's no way I could find a solid hour, or even thirty minutes, to dedicate to exercise.

When you find yourself in this situation, be careful. It would be easy to start using a crowded calendar as an excuse to get off track. If you miss even one or two workouts, you risk losing momentum and moving the whole fitness thing to the back burner. Discipline is something you must practice to possess. You don't become a disciplined person without sticking to a commitment when it's the least convenient and the most difficult thing to fit in.

Valid excuses are always available. In your day to day life, there will be a sick child to tend to, a birthday party to go to, or laundry trying to take over your home. Just remember that exercise has the added benefit of delivering mental focus. So by taking the time to fit in a workout, you'll have a better perspective for dealing with the rest of your life.

The last thing I'll say it this: if all you can find one day is ten minutes, go for it! Just be sure to make it a solid, all-out, no-holds-barred workout. The fact that you showed up even for ten minutes will drive home your commitment.

The Seventh Commandment

Results are a measure of personal progress.

At some point in the process of transforming your body, you may find that no matter what you try, you can't seem to make your thighs smaller or your stomach flatter. It may not be your imagination. Results are relative to you and your body type. Not everyone can have long, lean-looking legs and washboard stomachs. Your frame is unique, and you have to be realistic about the results you can expect.

If you've set out on the One-Day Way program to be your best each day and you've determined weight-loss goals you're working toward, allow your body to follow accordingly. Stop looking at the young woman on the stair climber next to you at the gym. Don't start wishing you could have her figure. And definitely don't buy magazines at the grocery store checkout if your self-esteem is worse after reading them. Your body is beautiful and perfectly flawed. Everyone's is. Work out with the knowledge that you're trying to achieve maximum results for *you*!

The Eighth Commandment

Strength training three times a week is essential.

Strength training has too many benefits to list all of them here, but I want to give you the most important ones. Strength training builds and maintains muscle, and muscle tissue protects your joints and bones. Part of the aging process is that once we hit our midtwenties, we all lose some muscle each year. Adding regular resistance training will combat this and keep you feeling youthful.

Also, muscle needs to be fed more frequently than fat. It's the backbone of our metabolism. Therefore, by developing lean muscle, you create a furnace that needs fuel. The more lean muscle you have compared to body fat, the faster your metabolism will work. The One-Day Way includes a commitment to strength training three times per week. Which days you do it is up to you. However, you'll receive the maximum benefit when you have a day off in between. Doing strength training every other day is optimal. If you're concerned about learning how to use complicated equipment or heavy weights, don't worry. In the next chapter you'll find the One-Day Way strength-training workout. I've designed it to deliver maximum results using simple strength-training equipment. I can't wait to show it to you!

The Ninth Commandment
Recovery is required.

Even God rested on the seventh day! When I began to exercise, I was much more concerned with making it stick than with the quality of the workout itself. I made sure I went to the gym six days in a row. But no matter what, I always took off the seventh day. Now my workouts are five or six days a week, depending on my schedule. But I still make time for recovery. Recovery rejuvenates your mind and your body. If you never take time off from working out, eventually it will feel more like "have to" instead of "get to." You don't want to approach exercise as an obligation or a duty. In truth, it is a privilege to have a body you can exercise. Keep this in mind as you schedule time off. And remember, your body will be stronger in the long run because you take a weekly break.

The Tenth Commandment
Figure out how to love exercise.

My husband, Keith, hates going to the dentist, especially to get his teeth cleaned. He says the scraping and picking drives him insane. My view of going to the dentist is entirely different. I like the feeling of clean teeth. I like leaving with that minty-fresh feeling. I think I even smile bigger and brighter for the next few days. But Keith recently went an extended period of time without seeing the dentist because he detests it so much. When he finally went, the cleaning was painful because he had put it off for too long.

The same principle of cause and effect applies to your workouts. If you can't find a way to enjoy exercising, you'll put it off and miss the benefits. And if you put it off, it can be painful to go back. By finding a way to like it, you can clearly see how the benefits outweigh whatever you don't like. Most people who tell me they don't like exercise are too results driven. If they can't see five pounds come off after a week's workout, they think, *What's the point?* The point is simply to show up today. And keep showing up, one day at a time.

If you dread walking on a treadmill, then get on some other piece of cardio equipment, or go outside and start jogging in a beautiful park. Some people need to have a ball involved in their cardio exercise to keep from getting bored. Great! This means you should never be at a loss. You can choose from tennis, racquetball, basketball, and many others. Weight loss and muscle tone will be a by-product if you figure out a way to like exercise.

A FEW CARDIO SUGGESTIONS

Basketball	Recumbent bike/bicycling outdoors
Boxing/sparring	Rollerblading
Brisk walking	Running
Cross-country skiing	Snowboarding
Dancing	Soccer
Elliptical machine	Spinning
Football	Stair climber
Hockey	Step aerobics
Ice-skating	Swimming
Kick boxing	Tennis
Racquetball	Water aerobics

· ·

Chapter 15

The One-Day Way Strength-Training Workout

All You Need Is One Band, One Ball

I am excited about introducing the One-Day Way strength-training workout! Not only will it strengthen and tone your entire body, but it's also fun. And you won't need to buy lots of fancy, expensive equipment. The One-Day Way strength exercises are built around two simple pieces of equipment: a medicine ball and a resistance band. One ball, one band, that's it!

My good friend Denise, whose story you read at the end of chapter 7, helped me design this strength-training program. Denise and I both know from experience how to take off weight, transform our bodies, and teach others to do the same. We also know that the best form of training comes from functionality. This means you'll be strengthening the parts of your body that you use every day in gardening, moving boxes, or dusting a ceiling fan. You'll work on muscles that you use to stand on a ladder and clean windows, remove a spare tire from your car, scrub baseboards, and lug groceries with a baby on your hip. All these ordinary life activities require strength, flexibility, and muscle tone. As you work against the weighted medicine ball and the resistance band, you'll be toning your core muscles (those in your torso), improving flexibility, and building overall strength.

WHY THE MEDICINE BALL AND RESISTANCE BAND?

Medicine balls have been used for generations to build strength. During World War I medics on troop ships would stuff rags into leather basketballs to give injured soldiers something weighted to throw around as a way to help them recover faster. Today many athletes and fitness experts consider medicine balls to be fantastic tools for core conditioning and building physical strength.

A medicine ball is more versatile than you may think. You can throw it, catch it, chase it. You can incorporate the ball into movements using several body parts at one time. And remember, when you engage a number of muscles at the same time, you get an intense cardio workout as well. This happens because your heart must work harder to supply energy to all the muscle groups being engaged. If you're a multitasker, you'll appreciate the benefit of exercising a number of body parts simultaneously.

I'm sure you've heard the saying that you are only as strong as your weakest link. The number-one reason for injuries such as torn ligaments, sprains, and strains is weak muscles surrounding the joints in our bodies. I'll teach you exercises with the medicine ball that will condition your entire musculature. This will happen because we eliminate the fixed motions of stationary weight machines and replace them with explosive and repetitious real-life movements.

Medicine balls come in various sizes, weights, and styles. Some even bounce, although the exercises in this book do not require that. If you haven't had much experience with strength training, I recommend starting with a six- to eight-pound ball. Once you've worked out with the ball for a few months, you might consider purchasing one that is heavier, to add more challenge.

In addition to the medicine ball, the exercises at the end of this chapter use a resistance band. The beauty of the band is that it provides resistance with a full range of motion. Exercise bands generally provide a certain degree of resistance—light, medium, or heavy. If you're just beginning, I recommend you start with a light or medium band. You can always get a thicker and more challenging band down the road.

The simplicity of the One-Day Way fitness system carries through to strength training. You don't need to learn about free weights or exercise machines. You don't have to worry about which body parts you train. Instead, you can simply focus on being fit each day!

I know firsthand how overwhelming it can be to go from a nonexistent or limited workout schedule to five days of cardio and three days of strength training each week. So start out with a simple commitment: For the first week, begin each day with the pledge to break a sweat by doing cardio exercise. Beginning with the second week, learn and complete only one strength-training exercise from this book every day. In less than five weeks, you will have tried and learned all thirty-one exercises in this chapter.

Once you've learned them all, you'll be about six weeks into your One-Day Way of life. At that point you should include three strength-training sessions in your workouts every week. Because you spent the previous weeks familiarizing yourself with all thirty-one exercises, choose five or six to complete for each workout. Then rotate them regularly. What you build your body to look like is up to you. These are the tools and building materials to do it!

ONE BALL, ONE BAND: THE ONE-DAY WAY TO GET STRONG

Here are the thirty-one strength-training exercises.

1. Sit-ups with Ball Toss . . . .

1. Lie on your back with knees bent up and feet flat on the floor. Grip the medicine ball so it's touching your chest.

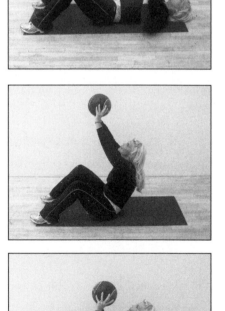

2. Holding the ball against your chest, sit up slowly. When your torso is perpendicular to the floor, toss the ball into the air and catch it.

3. Bring it back to your chest. Slowly lie down flat, back into the starting position.

Do three sets. First set, twenty repetitions. Second set, fifteen repetitions. Third set, ten repetitions.

2. Pull-over with Leg Vs •

1. Lie flat on your back, holding the medicine ball with both hands and your arms extended straight out on the floor behind your head. Extend your legs in a V shape on the floor.

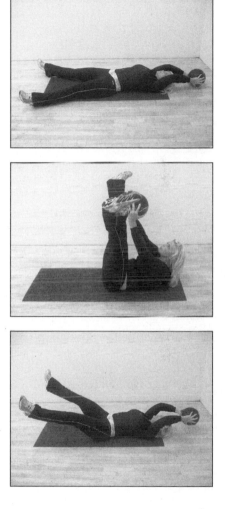

2. Form a triangle with your body by lifting the ball and your legs until they meet above your midsection.

3. Return slowly to your starting position. Maintain the V shape with your legs, keeping your arms and legs straight.

Do three sets of fifteen repetitions. Rest fifteen seconds between sets.

3. Triceps Extension with Static Leg Hold • • • • • • • • • • •

1. Lie flat on your back, cross your feet at the ankles, and lift your legs to a 45-degree angle. Hold that position.

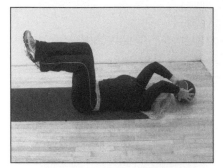

2. Holding the medicine ball in both hands, lift it directly above your chest with both arms fully extended.

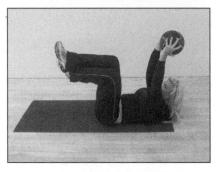

3. Bend your elbows and lower the ball to the floor just behind your head. Then raise your arms and push the ball upward so it is again positioned above your chest.

Do five sets of twenty repetitions each.

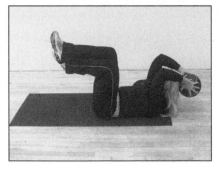

4. Front Kick with Ball Press • • • • • • • • • • • • • • • • • •

1. Stand with your feet shoulder width apart. Hold the ball in both hands with your elbows bent and your arms close to the sides of your body.

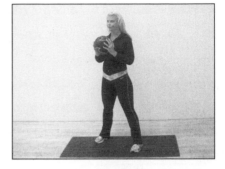

2. Press the ball away from your chest while kicking your right leg forward. Kick as high as you can.

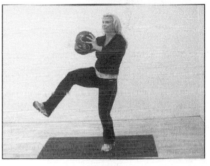

3. Bring the ball back down to chest level, while continuing to kick.

For one set, do fifteen kicks with the right leg, then fifteen kicks with the left leg. Repeat for a total of two sets.

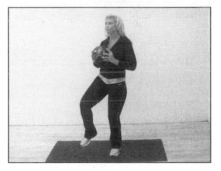

5. Band Squat with Back Row . . . .

1. Place a resistance band under your feet, and stand with your feet shoulder width apart and your knees slightly bent. In each hand take hold of one of the ends of the resistance band. (To ensure the band is taut enough to provide sufficient resistance, you may need to wrap it around your hands once.)

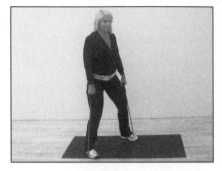

2. Bend your knees into a squat, going no lower than having your thighs parallel to the floor and keeping your back as straight and upright as possible.

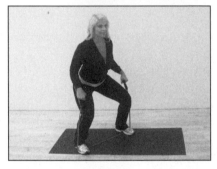

3. Stand back up, pressing your chest out and pulling the band upward and backward until your hands are at shoulder height. Hold the row (pull) for ten seconds.

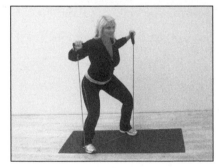

Do three sets of fifteen repetitions.

6. Sumo Band Squat with Shoulder Press • • • • • • • • • • • •

1. Stand with your feet farther than shoulder width apart, toes aimed slightly outward in a sumo wrestler type stance. Place the center of the band under your feet and hold the ends thigh high.

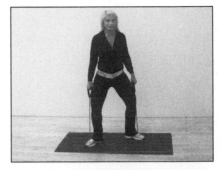

2. Squat until your knees are bent at a 45-degree angle. Keep your back straight and your knees bent so your knees line up over the center of your feet.

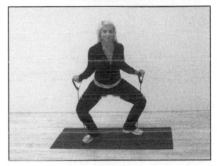

3. Stand back up by straightening your knees. At the same time pull the band straight above your head until your arms are fully extended.

Do three sets. First set, twenty repetitions. Second set, fifteen repetitions. Third set, ten repetitions.

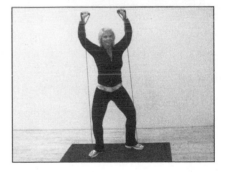

7. Throw Back, Go Fetch . . . .

1. Standing with your legs hip distance apart, bend your knees slightly, and hold the medicine ball below waist level, allowing it to touch your thighs.

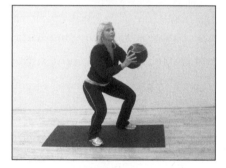

2. Squat down with your back straight, then swing the ball up and over your head, and throw it behind you.

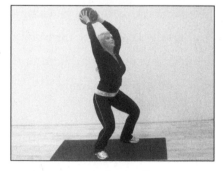

3. Turn around and fetch the ball. Bring it back to the starting position.

Do three sets of ten repetitions.

8. Frog Leap with Ball Throw Down • • • • • • • • • • • • •

1. Stand with your feet farther apart than shoulder width, toes pointed slightly outward. Grip the ball in both hands with your arms held out in front of you.

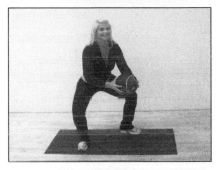

2. Squat, then leap up like a frog while extending both arms above your head.

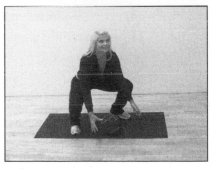

3. While you're coming down, throw the ball to the floor. Pick it up, and go back to the starting position to repeat.

Do two sets of fifteen leaps. Rest two minutes between sets.

9. Wall-Ball Push-up with One Leg . . . .

1. While standing, extend your arms in front of you, and place the ball against a wall. Hold the ball on both sides with your hands while stepping backward, away from the wall.

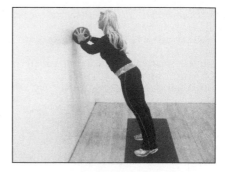

2. Bending your elbows, press your body weight into the ball and extend your left leg behind you.

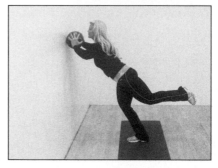

3. Straighten your arms to push away from the wall while continuing to extend your left leg behind you.

Do three sets of ten repetitions on each leg.

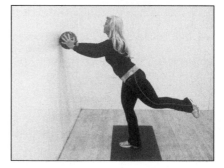

10. Band Sit-ups with Shoulder Press ● ● ● ● ● ● ● ● ● ● ● ● ●

1. Sit on the floor with your knees bent, and place the center of the band underneath your bottom. Hold the ends of the band in front of you with your elbows down to your sides.

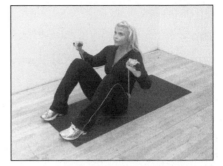

2. While tightening your abdominals, lower your body backward until your entire back brushes the floor.

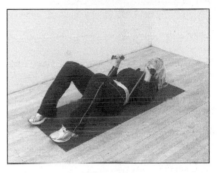

3. As you raise your torso back up and return to your original position, resist the band and press your hands toward the ceiling.

Do three sets of fifteen repetitions.

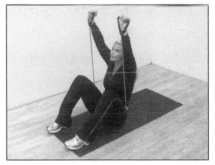

11. Seated Ball Chest Press · · · · · · · · · · · · · · · · · ·

1. Sit on the floor with your back straight, your shoulders pulled back, and your legs flat against the floor in a V shape.

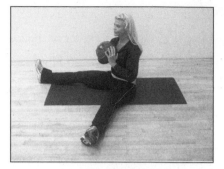

2. Hold the ball at the center of your chest, and squeeze it with both hands.

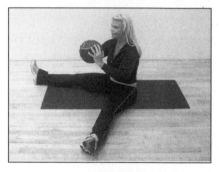

3. Push the ball straight out in front of you while tightening your chest muscles. Hold your arms straight out at shoulder height for ten seconds, then bring the ball back to your chest.

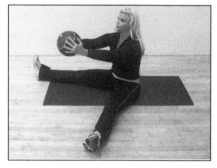

Repeat for five sets of ten repetitions.

12. Straight-Leg Dead Lifts with Ball • • • • • • • • • • • • •

1. Stand with your feet shoulder width apart, and hold the ball, with both hands, against your thighs.

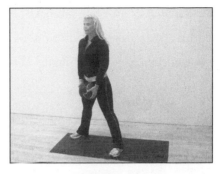

2. Keeping your knees straight, bend forward at the waist, and bring the ball as close to the floor as you can.

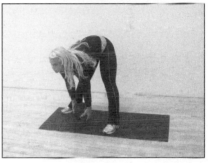

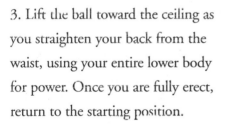

3. Lift the ball toward the ceiling as you straighten your back from the waist, using your entire lower body for power. Once you are fully erect, return to the starting position.

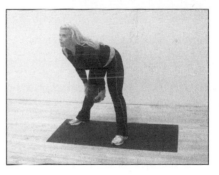

Do three sets of fifteen repetitions.

13. Around-the-World Ball Rotations • • • • • • • • • • • •

1. Stand with your feet shoulder width apart. Hold the ball close to your chest but not touching.

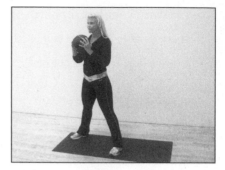

2. With your back straight, extend your arms to the left, then swing the ball overhead and then down to the right in a wide, high arc with your arms fully extended. Continue making a full circle, until your arms are straight down at knee height. Bring the ball back up to the starting position at the center of your chest.

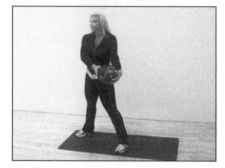

Repeat in a clockwise rotation for two sets of twenty rotations, then rest for two minutes. Repeat in a counter-clockwise direction for two sets of twenty rotations.

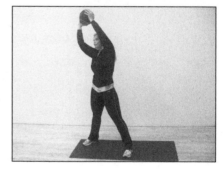

14. Side Lunge with Batter's Swing • • • • • • • • • • • • • •

1. Stand with your feet farther apart than shoulder width. With your arms straight, hold the medicine ball in both hands and point it toward the floor.

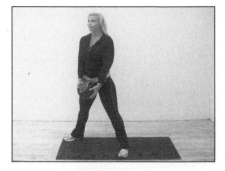

2. Step out to your right side into a side lunge with both feet pointing forward. (Hop to the side using both legs.) While you lunge to the right, raise the ball to the right as high as you can. Then swing the ball down until it touches your right thigh.

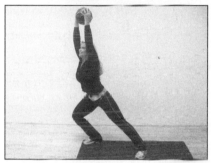

3. Hold the lunge and swing the ball up to the left side until both arms are fully extended toward the ceiling. Return to the starting position.

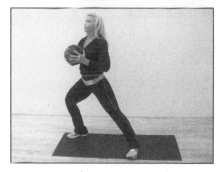

Repeat for two sets of fifteen repetitions on each side. Rest for one minute between sets.

15. Ball Transfer with Squat . . . .

1. Stand with legs no more than hip distance apart. Grip the ball with both hands, and hold it chest high.

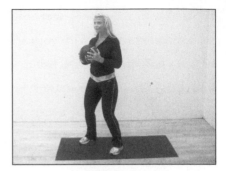

2. Place the ball between the centers of your thighs, and use your leg muscles to hold it in place. With arms raised straight out in front of you, begin to squat down while keeping the ball locked between your legs.

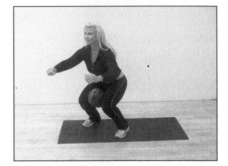

3. Stand up, and bring the ball back to the starting position.

Do three sets of fifteen repetitions. Rest for thirty seconds between sets.

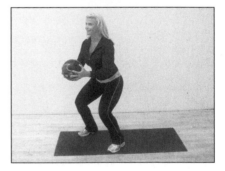

16. Lying Leg Scissors • • • • • • • • • • • • • • • • • • •

1. Lie on your back on the floor. Lift your legs straight up with your knees touching, and place the resistance band across the soles of your feet. Then wrap the ends of the band around each hand once.

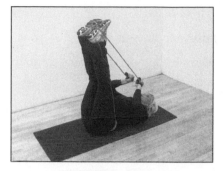

2. Separate your legs into a V shape while pulling the band toward the floor beside your shoulders.

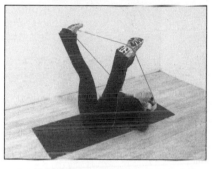

3. Move your legs together and apart in a scissorlike movement while holding the ends of the band just above your shoulders.

Do three sets of twenty "scissor cuts." Rest one minute. Then do three sets of thirty.

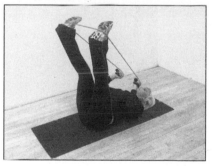

17. Lying Band Quad Press . . . .

1. Lie on your back, and bring your knees up to your chest. Keep your feet side by side, and place the band across the center of your soles. Wrap each end of the band one time around your hands.

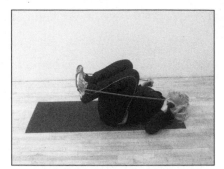

2. Straighten your legs out parallel to the floor, pushing your feet away from your body, while holding the ends of the band next to your shoulders.

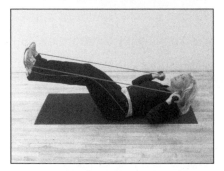

3. Pull your knees back in toward your chest, then straighten out your legs again.

Do three sets of twenty repetitions.

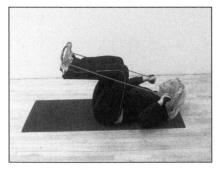

18. Single Straight-Leg Extension • • • • • • • • • • • • •

1. Lie on your back with your right knee bent at a 45-degree angle. Keep your left leg flat on the floor with the band placed across the sole of your foot. Wrap the ends of the band once around each hand.

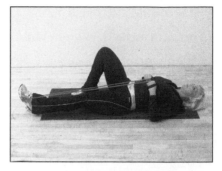

2. Raise your left leg off the floor by pulling the band up, then pulling it toward your chest.

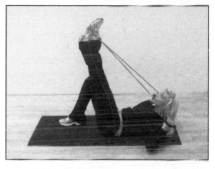

3. Continue to raise your left leg and bring the left knee in to touch your chest. Then straighten and lower your left leg to the starting position. Repeat steps 1 through 3 using your right leg.

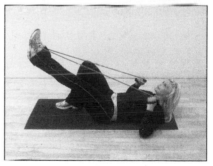

Do three sets of fifteen repetitions on each side.

19. Ball Planks . . . .

1. Kneel with both knees on the floor. Lean forward, and put both hands on top of the medicine ball.

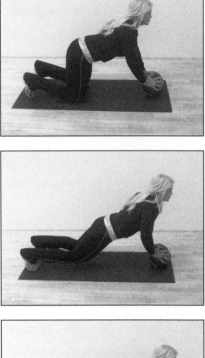

2. With both hands gripping the ball, straighten your arms. Then straighten your legs by supporting yourself on your toes, raising your knees off the floor, and stepping backward.

3. Continue stepping back until your legs and back form a straight line. While keeping your elbows locked, hold the position and focus on tightening your abdominal and chest muscles.

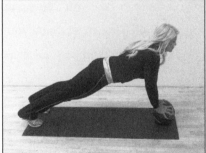

First set, hold for fifteen seconds. Second set, hold for twenty seconds. Third set, hold for thirty seconds.

20. Hands-on-Ball Kickback • • • • • • • • • • • • • • • •

1. Kneel with both knees on the floor. Lean forward, and put your hands on the medicine ball.

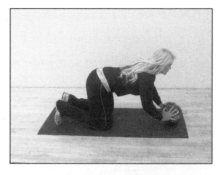

2. Keep your left knee resting on the floor. Pull your right knee upward toward your chest while bending your arms and lowering yourself down into the ball (as if doing a push-up). Hold for ten seconds.

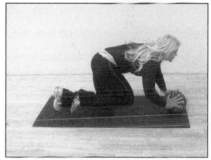

3. Kick back with your right leg, raising it as high as possible, and hold the position for ten seconds. Put your right knee back on the floor. Repeat the steps with your left leg.

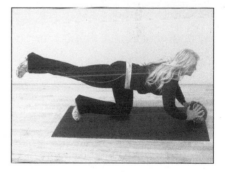

Do three sets of fifteen repetitions. Rest one minute between sets.

21. Hands on Side Plank . . . .

1. Lie on your right side, leaning on your right forearm. Hold the ball directly out in front of you with it resting on the floor.

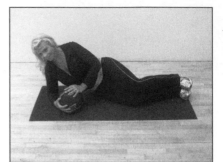

2. Keep your feet together and your legs and back in a straight line. Lift your body off the ground, using your left arm. (You are pulling up with your oblique muscles.)

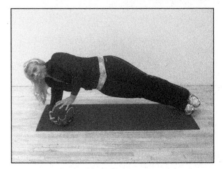

3. Lower your body toward the floor without touching it. Raise your body and repeat. (This exercise is similar to a one-arm push-up from the side.)

Do three sets of ten repetitions on each side.

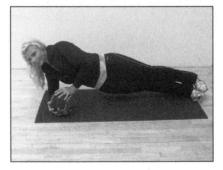

22. Side-Plank Hip Lift with Static Ball Hold • • • • • • • • • •

1. Lie on your right side, resting on your right hand. Grip the ball with your left hand.

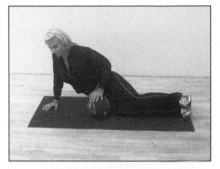

2. Straighten your left arm, and begin to raise your body by pushing upward with your hips. Hold ten seconds in this position.

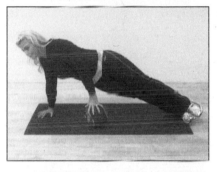

3. Next, lower your body halfway, and hold for ten seconds.

Do fifteen repetitions with a ten-second hold for each position. Then repeat on the left side.

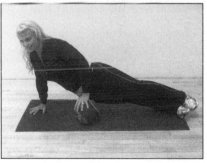

23. Seated Curl, Press, Extension • • • • • • • • • • • • • • • • •

1. Sit on the floor with your back straight and your legs flat on the floor and open to a V. Keeping your abdominals tight, grip the ball with both hands, and hold it out in front of you.

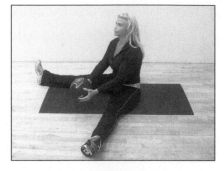

2. Lower the ball until it touches the floor between your legs. Keeping your elbows close to your sides, bend your arms at the elbow to raise (curl) the ball upward.

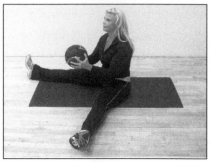

3. Then raise the ball overhead. While keeping your arms close to the sides of your head, bring the ball back down in front of your chest and then curl it back up. Return the ball to the starting position.

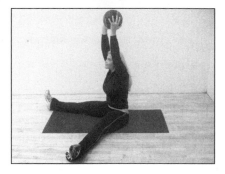

Do three sets of fifteen repetitions.

24. Seated Forward Reach • • • • • • • • • • • • • • • • • •

1. Sit on the floor with your back straight and your legs open to a V. Grip the ball with both hands and raise it to chest height. Bring the ball in to touch your chest.

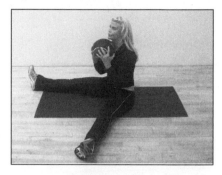

2. Push the ball away from your chest, reaching forward with your arms, extending them as far as you can, and keeping them parallel to the floor. Hold that position for five seconds, taking in a deep breath.

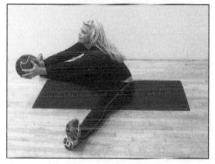

3. Exhale, then bring the ball back to your chest. Straighten your back as you return to the starting position.

Do three sets of ten repetitions.

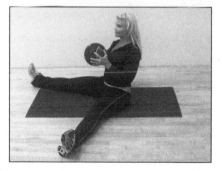

25. Seated Ball Chest Squeeze with Side Bend . . . .

1. Sit on the floor with your back straight and your legs straight and open in a V. Hold the ball with both hands at chest level and squeeze it.

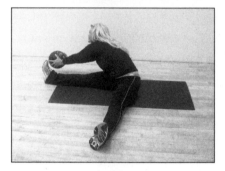

2. Bend from the waist to the right side while extending the ball away from your chest and toward your right foot.

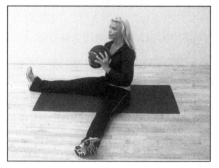

3. Pull the ball back to your chest, squeeze it, and repeat steps one and two going toward your left foot.

Do three sets of fifteen repetitions, extending the ball first toward your right foot, then toward your left foot.

26. Ball Crawl. •

1. Kneel on the floor, and place the ball in front of you on the floor. Bend at the waist at a 45-degree angle, keeping your back straight.

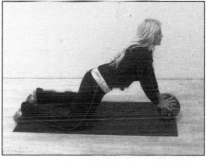

2. While alternating hands, roll the ball forward, keeping your arms straight, until your legs are at a 45-degree angle.

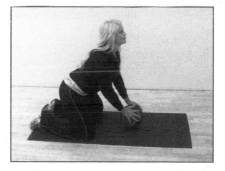

3. Then roll the ball back toward your knees, alternating hands, until you return to the starting position.

Repeat the crawl ten times.

27. Static Ball Press with Bicycle Extension . . . .

1. Lie flat on your back on the floor. Bring both knees up so that your legs are at a 90-degree angle. Keep your hips on the floor.

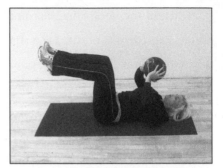

2. Grip the medicine ball with both hands, and push it up until your arms are above you as shown in the picture. While continuing to hold the ball, extend your legs back and forth, as if pedaling a bicycle.

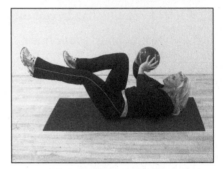

3. Lower the ball, and return to the starting position.

First set, pedal for twenty seconds. Second set, thirty seconds. Third set, forty seconds.

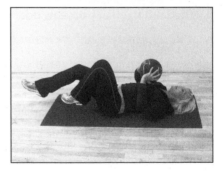

28. Doorknob Band Jabs •

1. Wrap the middle of a band around a doorknob a few times, making sure it's secure and the loose ends are an equal length. Turn your back to the door, standing between the two strands and holding one end in each hand.

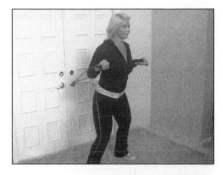

2. Take a step forward and lean your upper body until you feel a strong amount of resistance.

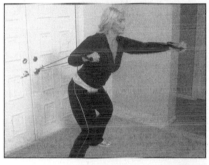

3. Keep your hands in front of you. As if boxing, jab (punch) forward, alternating right and left hands.

Do five one-minute segments of jabs with a thirty-second rest between segments.

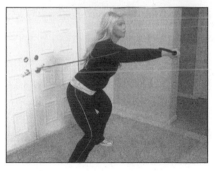

29. Doorknob, Biceps, Static Squat . . . .

1. Wrap the center of the resistance band around a doorknob a few times, making sure that it's secure and that the loose ends are an equal length. Face the door, and hold one end of the band in each hand.

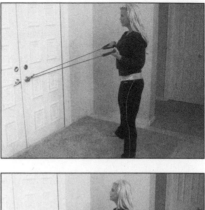

2. Take a few steps backward. With your feet shoulder width apart, squat, keeping your back straight and making sure your knees don't go beyond your toes. Hold that position for a fifteen-second count.

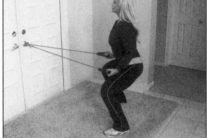

3. Hold the band with palms facing forward. Use both hands to lower it thigh high, keeping your elbows tight to your sides. Begin curling the band until your hands are at your shoulders. Hold the band at the highest point for five seconds, then release the tension.

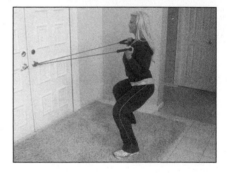

Repeat the steps for three sets of fifteen repetitions each.

30. Doorknob Chest Fly, Static Lunge · · · · · · · · · · · · · · · ·

1. Wrap the center of the band around a doorknob a few times, making sure it's secure and the ends are an equal length. Stand facing the door. With an end of the band in each hand, hold your arms straight in front of you at chest level.

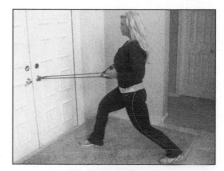

2. Take a small step forward with your right leg, and lunge with your left until it nearly touches the floor. Hold this position for a count of fifteen seconds.

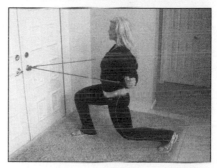

3. With your palms facing each other, pull your hands straight back until your elbows go beyond your back.

Do three sets of twenty repetitions.

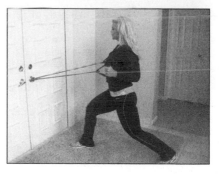

31. Doorknob Oblique Pull and Side Lunge . . . .

1. Wrap the center of the band around a doorknob a few times, making sure it's secure and the ends are an equal length. Turn your body so your right side is facing the door.

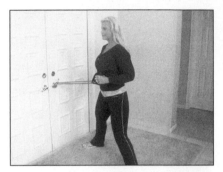

2. Step away from the door, holding both strands of the band with your left hand and pulling the band across your waist, while lunging to your side. Stand far enough away from the door that you have strong resistance from the band.

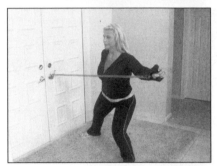

3. Extend your left arm away from your side and keep it straight. Raise it to shoulder height while pivoting away from the wall and increasing the band's resistance.

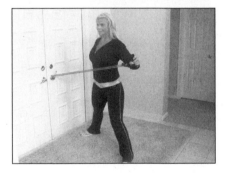

Do three sets of twenty repetitions on each side.

. . . .

PART 4

Your Road to Completion

How to Develop Lasting Power

. . . .

Chapter 16

The Power of Protection

You Need to Safeguard
Your New Life

When Keith and I had our first child, I was amazed at how much equipment one little baby needed. From bottles and pacifiers to big things like strollers and bassinets. The bag I used for hauling all of my baby's stuff was bigger than any purse I'd ever owned. I soon realized that while most of the equipment was necessary, some of it was not. Really, do we need a wipe warmer? Or those videos that supposedly make an infant smarter?

But parents can't be without a car seat during their child's early years. And once a child starts crawling, many parents—especially those who live in homes with more than one level—waste no time installing a baby gate. Car seats, baby gates, and baby latches on cabinet doors all provide a measure of protection to keep your baby safe from danger.

You and I need protection as well. As we build our new lives, we have to think about the things that can potentially endanger our achievements. Even though you're committed to losing weight, becoming fit, and living better all around, everything can be destroyed in an instant. Even if you have established a solid foundation and have begun to implement a new attitude and outlook, you're still susceptible to hazardous conditions. That's why we need to talk about protection.

In a community that has suffered a rash of break-ins, everyone in the neighborhood wants to avoid being the next victim. Homeowners install alarm systems. I remember the time I had a security company come out to give me a quote. The sales rep's primary goal is to sell the homeowner the best (meaning the most expensive) security system he can. His method is to try to scare the potential buyer. He wants you to think that if you don't wire every window and door in your house, you will most certainly regret it.

After listening to his high-pressure sales pitch, you're certain that if you don't sign on the dotted line, you'll be robbed of everything you hold near and dear. You see visions of your home as a crime scene and of yourself setting out on a wild-goose chase, visiting pawn shops in search of the watch Grandpa left you in his will.

Are scare tactics effective? For some people. But others don't buy into them. They choose to live on the edge, betting they'll beat the odds. They decide to live without a security system, choosing not to live in fear.

Others might want to have more protection, but they can't afford it. Even though they're afraid, they have faith that no one will break into their house. This approach can be costly, because sometimes faith won't stop a thief. And then there are those who sign up but never schedule the appointment to install the system. Perhaps the fear of being the next victim was soon forgotten. For whatever reason, the security system was never put in. As a result their house is a target because it's unprotected.

PROTECTING YOUR NEW LIFE

Your desire for a new life needs to be protected. You should be safe to dream big and to succeed in accomplishing your goals. That's why you need a personal alarm system to guard your hopes and dreams.

How do you do that? Here's what has worked for me and countless other people I've coached: put your commitment in writing before you begin. It's true that the One-Day Way is all about living and achieving one day at a time. Therefore, regular recordkeeping is forbidden. (If you lost a half pound yesterday, that's great. But what are you doing *today* to build your new life?) Focusing on counting your successes and recording your incremental progress will sabotage the purpose of the plan, because you'll think success can't happen today but only in the distant future. You'll grow discouraged by any little slip-up. Or you'll lose interest because "real progress" seems to be taking way too long.

So don't keep records. If you write in a fitness journal, tear today's page out tomorrow and discard it. However, there is great value in committing to a *binding contract,* a personal agreement that states your full intentions to turn your convictions into reality.

I'll tell you a somewhat-embarrassing story that happened recently. In my first book, *Never Say Diet,* I included two suggestions for readers. One was to create a personal-surrender statement. The reader was to write a few sentences that expressed her commitment to the program and her willingness to let go of the past. I suggested that readers memorize their statement and recite it each day. The second suggestion involved the Brain Change Contract, which is similar to the agreement you'll find later in this chapter. It spells out your commitment to live each day fully committed to the mission of being the best you can be. Both statements included in *Never Say Diet* were meant to be signed by the reader and witnessed by a friend.

After I'd done my radio show one day, a station employee brought his wife to meet me. She had read *Never Say Diet* and asked me to autograph her copy. She also wanted me to witness her surrender statement, a personally created promise to build a new life, according to my suggestion in *Never Say Diet*.

I was thrilled to meet this beautiful woman. We connected and began to chat. Next she pulled out a folder with a sheet of paper inside. She asked, "Would you please sign this?" It had been nearly two years since I'd written *Never Say Diet*. But this woman had read the book only a couple of weeks earlier. The idea behind the personal-surrender statement was fresh in her mind but not in mine.

So I told her in a kidding way, "I need to read this first if I'm going to sign it." We laughed, and I began to read. Without looking up, I told her, "Wow, great job of writing this! It's really awesome. It's exactly what you need to be thinking. I'll gladly witness this. Let's never forget what a tremendous moment in your life this is going to be!" As I looked up and tried to convey how impressed I was, she looked away and said, "I'm really glad you feel this way about your own work."

She had decided to use my Brain Change Contract (verbatim from my book) as her personal surrender statement. It's fine to do that, but I had misunderstood. So without meaning to, I was letting her know how incredibly impressed I was with *my own words and work.*

Imagine getting out of that one! It wasn't easy. I explained how I'd been confused. Then we laughed and moved on. To this day she's probably wondering how often I get my hair colored blond and if the chemicals are damaging my brain. Truthfully, my mind is sometimes scattered. That's why I like to write down the things that are most important to me. That's why I included a written agreement in this book (see pages 194–95).

The One-Day Way Contract is something I want you to take seriously. Think of me, at this moment, as the home-security-system sales rep telling you a dire story about all the things that could go wrong. I want to do everything I can to help you succeed. I want to see you achieve your desire to change your life. I want you to be safe and to live well. However, I know how quickly things can go wrong. It's time for you to bind your desire, put up some protection, and show up for the appointment…every day.

Read the contract that follows, and ask yourself if you can affirm what it says. As you read through it, feel free to change a few things if you want to make it more personal. The point is to keep the signed statement close by so it will do what it's meant to do—protect you. Having an alarm installed is important. But if you don't arm it every time you enter and exit your home, it won't provide much protection. As it pertains to your new life, you have come too far to be robbed of even one day.

Do you want to move closer to fulfilling your destiny? Of course, losing weight will require work each day. Working out and moving your body must be a nonnegotiable part of life every day. This is why protection is a key to keeping your commitment locked up.

Below is the One-Day Way Contract. Find someone to privately witness it, ask him or her to keep you accountable to it, and promise not to get mad when that person asks how you're doing in the days to come. In fact, volunteer to let him or her know on a weekly basis. While this may feel uncomfortable, it will provide the needed protection as you begin to reconstruct your life.

THE ONE-DAY WAY CONTRACT

I am fully committed to reconstructing my life. I know that I am a true work in progress. However, I am willing to finally face the areas that have been falling apart for too long. I will take care of my body each day. This means I will eat quality food the majority of the time, and I will make the quantity match my weight-loss goals. I will exercise and won't complain about doing it. I am willing to find new ways of moving and to mix up my workouts so I feel challenged all the time.

I will build my faith each day, even when I don't feel strong. I know that having faith and practicing it will be a tie that binds my commitment to everything meaningful that I set out to do in life.

It is also my heart's desire to make a difference in the lives of others by encouraging them, never tearing them down.

I also commit to taking responsibility for my life and to valuing myself as a person who has been made valuable by my Creator. I am beautiful today. I have been created to have a purpose and a destiny. I will not make excuses or accept my shortcomings as reasons to continue feeling defeated. No matter how many times I've screwed up in the past, my old mistakes are behind me. They are irrelevant to the work I'm doing now.

From today forward I will recommit each day to beginning fresh. I will get over trying to count up days I have done really well. I will also stop believing the lie that my successes from yesterday matter.

What I know is this:

- One day at a time I will wake up, choose to live well this day, and choose to begin anew.

- One day at a time I will make my actions match my desires, all day. These include attaining a healthy weight and wearing the size clothing I feel most comfortable in. This also includes taking care of my body with regular movement, which I finally accept I was designed to do. Strength training is also a part of my life.

- One day at a time I will make it my mission to be the best I can be no matter what happens, no matter how overwhelmed I feel or how crowded my schedule becomes. I will change my life in spite of the demands and pressures of daily life.

- One day at a time I will begin to see every event that happens or has happened as part of a grander plan to propel me forward, even if it seems like an accident, a setback, or a screwup. Instead, I will consider it a serendipity and smile more.

- And finally, one day at a time I will remind myself that tomorrow's almost here, especially whenever I feel like I'm not making enough progress. I won't buy this lie. I am ready to reconstruct my life and protect my One-Day Way program.

I have let go of the past. I love my life, and I will live well for as long as I am meant to be on earth. My cup will be full each morning. I am ready to "roll" this way, every day, beginning today.

Signed: _____

Date: _____

Witnessed: _____

· · · · · · · · · · · · · · · · · · · ·

Chapter 17

The Power of Tomorrow

Today Is the Key, but Another Day Awaits You

When I was about ten years old, I entered a county-fair talent contest. I wore a cute little dress and performed the song "Tomorrow" from the musical *Annie*. My mom played the piano, and I sang my chubby little heart out. I remember feeling happy because I loved to sing. Of course, the fair's cotton candy, popcorn, and caramel apples may have also contributed to the glow in my heart.

> Tomorrow! tomorrow! I love yah, tomorrow!
> You're always a day away![6]

In the musical when the sweet little orphan belts out these words, she seems positive. But you can tell she's actually feeling hopeless. She's trying to have a positive attitude, but she really is searching for someone who will take her in and love her. She dreams of being adopted, but it seems that no one wants her. While I wasn't an orphan and, in fact, grew up in a loving family, I still know what that feels like. Do you? I'm sure you have people who care about you, but do you feel unconditionally protected and loved?

Read the lyrics again. They sum up a great outlook to have when you embark on the One-Day Way of living. No matter how low you may feel one day, the words of the song remind us that a new day is less than twenty-four hours away. This is an awesome outlook! Instead of worrying about tomorrow, you can look toward the future with hopeful anticipation. It's a shift in perspective that will keep you on course forever.

THE POWER OF THE PRESENT

Most people refuse to live in the present. They're either stuck in regrets about their past or consumed with worry about the future—or both! As a result they don't live in the moment. Their emotions are tied up elsewhere. They have nothing left to give to living their life today!

Tomorrow is a new day, but worrying about it can steal today's potential for celebration. Likewise, you need to let go of yesterday. Worrying about what happened a week ago (and continuing to beat yourself up over it) does nothing to help you build the life you desire.

When you dwell in the past too much, you may begin to think you can't change. You may believe that because you've always made certain choices and done things a certain way, you'll always continue to do so. Friend, that is called hopelessness. But you don't have to live that way. You can change your life!

I was in the checkout line at the grocery store when I saw a woman I knew from the gym. We started chatting. She confessed that no matter how hard she tried, she couldn't stop eating a bag of potato chips every day. In her cart I saw not one but three bags of chips. I thought, *It must be hard to resist eating chips if you're buying them three bags at a time.* But I didn't say anything.

Because we knew each other and she seemed to be looking for help, I told her to stop eating potato chips for just one day. I wasn't talking about forever. It would be a simple experiment, and tomorrow she would choose not to eat any chips. She had the power to decide not to do what she normally did. (Notice, I didn't tell her to put the bags of chips back on the shelf.)

She had developed a habit and practiced it for years. For her, the thought of not eating potato chips for one day was a daunting challenge. It follows that the idea of changing that habit forever would have seemed entirely impossible. So I challenged her to forgo the chips for just one day. Daunting, yet doable.

Imagine how I felt when, weeks later, she found me at the gym and told me she had given up potato chips the day after I'd seen her in the grocery store. And she had done it again the day after that. Feeling empowered, she had given up potato chips again the third day. After four days she had thrown them out entirely. And now she felt more in control of her cravings.

How cool is that?

If I had told my friend in the checkout line that she had to make a big plan to give up potato chips forever, she probably wouldn't have listened to me. Even if she'd agreed that a daily intake of potato chips was unhealthy and led to weight gain and even though my advice to give them up forever was based on truth, she would have felt it was unrealistic and impossible.

Or if I had condemned her by saying something like, "How could you eat a whole bag of chips by yourself?" she would have felt shame and anger. That kind of discouraging remark would have reinforced her belief that she couldn't change.

Instead, all I asked her to do was give up chips for one day. She did it the following day, and then that one day turned into another and another. Slowly she was changing her entire life.

The One-Day Way approach to living better and losing weight is all about remembering that no matter what, you can make it through a day at a time. You can give up potato chips (or maybe for you it's candy bars or cookies or pie) for just one day.

THE POWER OF TOMORROW

But this system is also meant to help you remember something else: no matter what, *tomorrow is almost here!* When you're in the midst of a discouraging, really tough day, instead of letting yourself lose strength, remember that tomorrow is just around the bend. I've found this helps me succeed in doing even small things. For example, if I really want an extra serving of breakfast cereal but know I shouldn't have it, I tell myself I can have more cereal—but *not today.* I can have some tomorrow. This perspective allows me to minimize the aggravation I feel at the moment. Instead of denying myself completely, I'm simply delaying gratification.

You will also gain strength in building your new life when you realize how much energy you once spent trying to keep up with your old desires. We've talked about how much easier it is to focus on a simple meal plan based on repeating the same healthy foods. We've talked about the simplicity of a daily, thirty-minute session of moving and sweating to strengthen your heart. And we've practiced thirty-one different exercises using a medicine ball and a resistance band for strength training.

The simple approach coupled with a focus on today will free up your concentration and will make extra energy available to you. No longer do you need to regret yesterday or worry about tomorrow or make elaborate plans for a six-month fitness regimen. So make the best use of the extra brain power you now have at your disposal.

And if you find that your initial goals weren't ambitious enough, the One-Day Way gives you the flexibility to rethink them. Now that you've increased your confidence, strength, faith, and hope, go ahead and set new goals. Build a new life that's even better than the one you used to imagine.

Likewise, if at first you set such lofty goals that they're dragging you down and making you feel defeated, revise them. What you want to accomplish overall needs to be reassessed and revamped all the time. Part of the One-Day Way is learning to adjust your priorities and then organizing your daily tasks accordingly.

As you work to become the best you can be, you can't plan further ahead than tomorrow, because your life, your circumstances, your challenges are always changing. What is the next step in reconstructing your life? That depends on what step you just took. It depends on what you need to work on, which is personal to your life. It will be different from what someone else needs to work on.

Something else that's exciting to think about is that tomorrow also signifies newness! Every day that you live the One-Day Way, you start with a full cup of energy, a positive attitude, inner strength, peace, patience, and perseverance. (Think of every new morning as a large can of Red Bull for your life.) By the time you get to the end of the day (or on tough days, by 10 a.m.), the glass filled with your "spark" is beginning to look empty. Conserving the energy you began the day with was not an option. You had to draw on the energy, patience, and strength when you needed it.

Since almost every day is challenging, by the end of the day, your glass is empty. But you never need worry that you won't have enough left to get you through your long list of future plans. Remember, tomorrow morning you get a *new* cup full of promise, hope, energy, and life. And tomorrow is almost here! When you open your eyes, a new glass will be filled to the top once again, just as it was the day before.

Here's a tip. Your cup can be full every morning if you will allow the God who created the sunrise to do the pouring. Try saying a simple prayer first thing, before your feet hit the floor. Ask God to fill your cup, to give you the energy and strength you need for this day. The strength He can give you surpasses anything you can get from an energy drink. And then, when the sun sets at the end of the day, pray a prayer of thanks.

The following morning everything you'll need for the next twenty-four hours will be there. The strength you'll need for tomorrow will be there tomorrow, not today. So wait for it. Revive. Renew. Be patient.

No Excuses, No Matter What Happens

Of course, there's also a downside to tomorrow. As you begin to make progress and achieve bite-size goals, tomorrow can become an excuse not to fully give your best today. Excuses are what hold most people back. In my book *Never Say Diet,* I address the top twenty excuses people use not to get healthy and fit. One of the first is a lack of time. Here's my response to that: you will *make* time for whatever you feel is important. Take, for example, scrapbooking. I love to look at finished scrapbooks. I can fully appreciate the time invested in cutting and gluing and adding cute stickers or creating funny captions for photographs. I have friends who spend entire weekends enjoying this pastime. They love it, so they find a way to get away from their family and work responsibilities to spend hours cropping and pasting.

We tend to get done the things we've decided are important. As you organize your day each morning, be sure to prioritize what you want to do. What is your bite-size goal for today? What one thing will you do in the area of faith, or food, or fitness? Just for today how can you be the best you can be? I don't want you to get to the end of the day and be tempted to beat yourself up for letting time slip through your fingers. Decide first thing each day what you will do to follow your desire to be your best.

If you don't make this decision each day, you'll stop moving forward. Pretty soon you'll be asking yourself, *Why can't I ever stick to anything?* Stick to it today, and realize that tomorrow will be here before you know it.

When I look back on the days of my personal journey, I can recall many of them being especially challenging. One that I mentioned in a previous chapter was the day I discovered I was pregnant with my fourth child. There I was, living one day at a time, one workout at a time, one meal at a time and having great success. I had already lost about 180 pounds. But I was not quite where I wanted to be, and I viewed pregnancy as an obstacle instead of a blessing. Certainly not because I didn't want another child but because I felt like my previous success at losing weight was going to be wasted. So I spent the entire day crying. I wasted many hours of a God-given day, upset about something that could possibly be the greatest news I'd ever receive.

When evening came, I sat down and had a long conversation with myself and God. I made some tough choices. The first being that I wasn't going to let this opportunity to carry a new life be overshadowed by my selfishness. Next, I would not let pregnancy be an excuse to let go of my day-to-day commitment to being the best I can be, which included regular exercise and healthy eating. Then I asked God for strength. When I woke up the next day, I worked out through a little morning sickness. That night I thanked God as I went to sleep. I was looking forward to both the uncertainty and the excitement of the next day.

Remembering that you'll have tomorrow can give you hope today. Especially when today is tougher than usual. When a dark cloud appears—and, trust me, it will—you have to believe that the sun is still there even though you can't see it. It's important not to get sidetracked with challenging circumstances. Instead, be empowered with the opportunity to rise above them!

Do you think Martin Luther King Jr. could have written the famous "I have a dream" speech if he'd focused on the circumstances of the day he was living in? He believed in a new and brighter forecast for tomorrow, and he did what he needed to do each day based on his dream. And because of his dream, much of what Dr. King pictured in the 1960s has now come to pass.

Tomorrow, and the hope for its arrival, can help us all have a clearer vision for today.

Chapter 18

The Power of Unpacking

Life Is Hard, but You Need to Dive In

K eith and I moved our family into a new home about a year and a half ago. The home we were saying good-bye to was the first home we owned. About two hours into moving day, I remembered a magazine article I'd read months before about the most stress-filled events one will ever experience in life. Moving was ranked in the top five, along with the death of a parent and losing a job. When I first read that, I thought it was an exaggeration. But trust me, I'm a full-blown believer today!

Everything associated with moving is full of so much emotion. It's difficult to process all that's going on. While there's the excitement of a new home to decorate and the anticipation of holidays and future fun times to be shared, there's also the sadness of saying good-bye to an old place. A place where the walls hold memories of many Thanksgivings gone by. And too many birthday candles to count.

When I looked at the front door of the house we were leaving, it stirred more memories than I could contain. I remembered the night, years before, when I ran through that door to wake up Keith. I had a big announcement: While driving home, I had just made the decision that I would lose weight, get healthy, and write books. Oh, the memory of the look on his face is still priceless to me even today. And now, weighing two hundred pounds less, I'm writing another book. Keith is still my biggest cheerleader.

This was where I brought little Luke home to meet his sisters, Ashley and Kayla, and his big bro, Jake. You may recall the story of Luke's arrival from earlier in this book when I introduced you to the power of seeing life from a serendipitous perspective. This home was filled with lots of serendipitous events. Sure, there were many stress-filled days that I'd rather forget, but there were many more days, thankfully, that were wonderful.

I also had to say good-bye to the living room where I sat with my firstborn daughter, Ashley, and explained to her about the birds and the bees. Just a few years earlier I had sat on the same sofa, going through *Teach Your Child to Read in 100 Easy Lessons* with her. The swimming pool in our backyard evoked memories of my son Jake learning to swim. And I remembered that just a few weeks into his lessons, I had called my mom to have her consider with me if perhaps my son was part amphibian. We lived on a cul-de-sac, and I remember the good beating it took from my sweet "mini-me," Kayla, as she practiced riding her bike without training wheels. She kept going until she perfected it. She's still persistent like that.

That home had the formal dining room where I entertained my grandparents for the last time with our children before both grandparents passed away. And I'll never forget Mom Hobbs (Keith's grandmother) tasting my Key lime pie in that room and asking if I fell asleep pouring in the lime juice. She smacked her lips to let me know it was a tad bitter. And the family roared with laughter.

None of us will forget the family room in that house. It will always be remembered as the gathering place for taco nights, pizza parties, and prayer time. But the most difficult part of the moving process for me is still hard to talk about. It was knowing my mom and dad wouldn't be living only a few doors away anymore. Yes, good times, great memories, lots of tears, and loads of laughter, all boxed up with our belongings and moved to a new house and a new season in our lives.

The move itself went pretty smoothly. We were able to handle it with the help of some family members. But, for me, the worst feelings arrived a few days later. Everything was unloaded but not unpacked. I looked around and felt so empty and lost. I was certain our new home was going to be great. It had lots more room, and it was a beautiful house. But the boxes seemed to be taking over. I didn't know where to begin. All I wanted was to be settled, to feel at home. It wasn't that I wanted to go back, but I realized our new life couldn't fully begin until we unpacked. I had to approach it one box at a time.

Moving In to Your New Life

I don't know what final straw made you pick up this book. Maybe there was no final straw. Perhaps you just thought it looked interesting. Maybe you don't know yet why you chose to read this book. But I believe it wasn't an accident. And I know why I wrote it. My purpose is to offer you the reassurance that your life doesn't need to feel cluttered and disorganized. If you're feeling that way, it's time to unpack and start living the One-Day Way. Boxes are meant to be a temporary holding place.

When we began the project of reconstructing your life, we started with demolition. You may recall that we talked about getting rid of your old ways of measuring success and about breaking down your goals into daily, bite-size pieces. I told you to demolish comparison thinking: to stop thinking you had to achieve someone else's goals or that you had to reach a friend-approved or spouse-influenced number on the scale before you could celebrate. Hopefully, you learned that celebrations are possible every single day.

Next, you prepared your mind and body by letting the dust settle and fasting for a day. Then you began to envision the new you, the person you are working to become, both inside and outside—in terms of losing weight and becoming fit. This was laying the foundation of your personal reconstruction.

And then the fun began as I introduced you to the One-Day Way system to have faith, to eat, and to be fit. You will have much more peace in your life each day if you'll find a balance in these three areas.

After destroying the old foundation, laying the new foundation, and building the structure, you have one thing left to do. Turn on the power, and move into your new life! I would guess you're a little nervous. Perhaps you're not sure if you have the right keys to unlock the front door. You could be second-guessing whether you know how to eat right or if you're doing the exercises correctly. This is normal. Most people want a guarantee about the future. And I'm sorry. The only guarantee will come in the form of a new day. Today holds great promise, and tomorrow isn't here yet, so don't tie up your energy worrying about it.

Then there's the issue of maintenance. What happens if the plumbing leaks or a tree limb falls on the roof? You may be wondering, *Can I really keep the weight off and keep up my workouts?* Again, yes you can! Just as you lost the weight and gained fitness, you'll choose to eat well and exercise every day as part of maintaining your new life. And trust me, even in a brand-new home, some things go wrong or need fixing. Maintenance is part of life. You'll deal with it as it comes, never forgetting that you've passed your point of no return.

So here we are. It's moving day. You must remember that no matter what each day holds, you can reorganize your body and your life, one day at a time. You will unpack one box at a time. There will always be lots of opportunities to second-guess yourself. This is why you need to get some bite-size, successful days under your belt right away. They'll make you believe that dealing with the stress of self-improvement and unpacking boxes is worth it.

Within a few weeks of moving into our new home, I was putting up a Christmas tree. The excitement of that first holiday season, as I hung the children's stockings by the fireplace, is with me still. But to create the memory, I first had to find the box with the ornaments and the treetop angel. Soon you'll have lots of successes and celebrations to recall. But like me, you must keep opening up boxes.

PREPARE NOW FOR THE CHALLENGES

Just when you feel as if you're really making progress and things start to seem more organized, something may happen to make you feel like packing up and moving out. You might seek comfort from the Häagen-Dazs company. Or even if you resist that temptation, you might begin to look for the wrong people to console you. Both can be dangerous. Don't let anyone pull you away from pursuing your goals.

Life is full of uncertainty and unforeseen circumstances. I can guarantee you'll be hurt and disappointed by someone you trust and love. And tomorrow an event could occur that will forever change who you are. Even if new, changing circumstances make you think that living the One-Day Way is impossible, you have the power within to choose to think differently. You can believe that even difficult circumstances have blessings attached. Don't forget: blessings can come from an accident, a screwup, or a seeming setback. How you view them is up to you.

I feel as though I've lived a pretty crazy life so far. I still pinch myself sometimes when I think about all the boxes I've packed and unpacked and repacked. Lots of the things I've experienced have been serendipities, but mainly my life has been a process of watching my God-given purpose unfold.

You may feel as though your life is in so many boxes at this moment that you don't know which one to open first. I've been there, and it can be overwhelming. Especially because the one that has your toothbrush in it didn't get labeled! But your desire to get a fresh start is why you need to jump right in, open one box, and start putting things away. Start today.

Are you ready to live in the new life you've built? Even though you may feel you have a long way to go in losing weight and becoming fit or rebuilding some relationship or area of your life, you can still live in your new life today. You now have all the power at your fingertips to flip on the light switch when you wake up every morning and say, "There's no place like home."

No matter where life leads, and no matter where we live or how many times we move, our real home is within. We have the opportunity every day to let go of old memories that hold us back. To build a new life today, you need to avoid worrying about next week and instead look forward to every tomorrow for a new start.

You can look forward to the rest of your life as a daily adventure, living one day at a time, each day full of the hope and potential to be better than the one before.

How to Find More Power

All the power you will ever need to heal from yesterday, live for today, and face tomorrow is available to you right now. The truest thing I've learned is that the only lasting source of strength in my life comes from God's love and His relentless pursuit of me. No matter what religion you are, and even if you've never believed in a higher being, today can be the day you choose to allow the God of the universe to take over and be your everything! If you've been running your own life based on your own wisdom and strength, you can continue doing that. But if there comes a day when you are so desperate for strength and help that you cry out to God, He will comfort you and give you peace.

Go to a quiet place, and humble yourself before Him. Get down on your knees, low to the ground, and just cry out. I promise, He will hear every word, He will catch every tear, and He will show you more compassion, mercy, and love than you have ever known.

For God so loved the world that he gave his one and only Son,
that whoever believes in him shall not perish but have eternal life.
(John 3:16)

I believe the One-Day Way will help you achieve the exciting goals you have for your life. I'd love to hear from you as it's happening. Please contact me at www.chantelhobbs.com. You can also use my Web site as a resource for further information or just to say hi!

Notes

. . . .

1. You can read more of my story in Chantel Hobbs, *Never Say Diet* (Colorado Springs: WaterBrook, 2007).
2. Proverbs 29:18, KJV.
3. See Hebrews 11:1.
4. See Hebrews 11:1.
5. "That's What Friends Are For," lyrics by Burt Bacharach and Carole Bayer Sager, Arista Records, 1982.
6. "Tomorrow," lyrics by Martin Charnin, Sony Classical/Columbia, 1977.

Introducing the One-Day Way Learning System

It's easy to read a book like this one and get excited about changing your life. But for most people, real-life drama—sick kids, work stress, relationship worries, you name it—will threaten to crowd out your best intentions.

But I have exciting news! If you truly believe great accomplishments are within reach, additional help is available. I created the One-Day Way Learning System to get you through those tough days. Check out www.chantelhobbs.tv to learn more about the special system that will reinforce the motivation and direction you received from reading this book. The learning system will help you on a practical level, making it possible to stick to your commitment to live better and be better each day.

You might also want to check out my Web site at www.chantel hobbs.com, where you will find music you can download to get you moving and having fun at the same time.

I am phenomenally blessed to be able to introduce you to the one-day approach to a new life. You can break bad habits and create good ones—and do it all in one day. Please don't spend another moment feeling frustrated and frazzled. Making the change is up to you.

You can dare to be remarkable right now!

Chantel

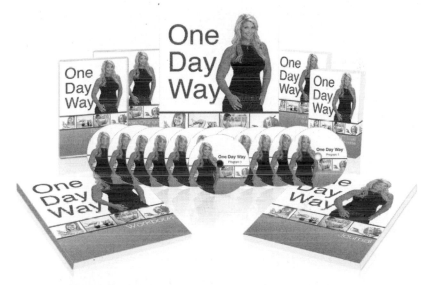
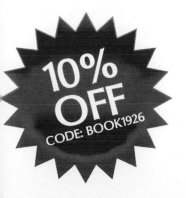

Put an end to the diet drama!

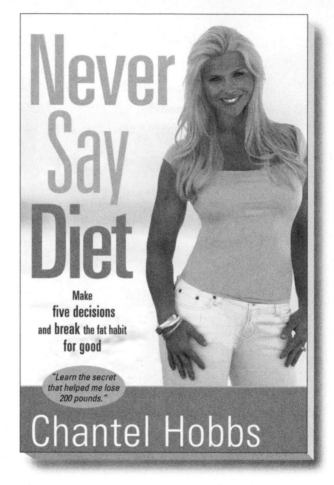

Ready to lose the frustration of up-and-down dieting? Discover five decisions that lead to permanent weight loss. Here is proof that when you change your mind you can change your life—for good.

www.ChantelHobbs.com

Available in bookstores and from online retailers.

WATERBROOK PRESS
www.waterbrookmultnomah.com